NCLEX-PN®
Maternal-Neonatal Nursing

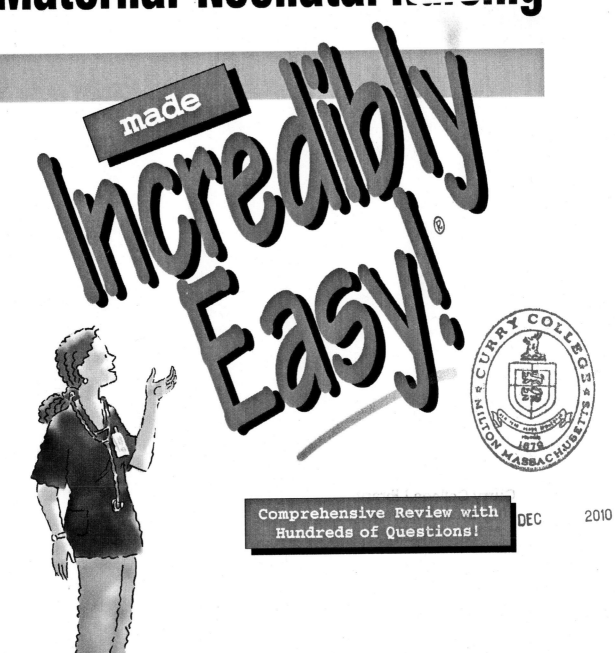

made Incredibly Easy!®

Comprehensive Review with Hundreds of Questions!

Wolters Kluwer | Lippincott Williams & Wilkins
Health

Philadelphia · Baltimore · New York · London
Buenos Aires · Hong Kong · Sydney · Tokyo

Staff

Publisher
Chris Burghardt

Clinical Director
Joan M. Robinson, RN, MSN

Clinical Project Manager
Beverly Ann Tscheschlog, RN, MS

Clinical Editor
Jennifer Meyering, RN, BSN, MS, CCRN

Acquisitions Editor
Bill Lamsback

Product Director
David Moreau

Product Managers
Rosanne Hallowell and Jennifer K. Forestieri

Editorial Assistants
Karen J. Kirk, Jeri O'Shea, Linda K. Ruhf

Art Director
Elaine Kasmer

Illustrator
Bot Roda

Vendor Manager
Cynthia Rudy

Manufacturing Manager
Beth J. Welsh

Production Services
SPi Technologies

Library of Congress Cataloging-in-Publication Data

ISBN-13: 978-1-4511-0818-7
ISBN-10: 1-4511-0818-4

Contents

Preface   *v*

Part I   Getting ready

1   Preparing for the NCLEX®   3
2   Strategies for success   15

Part II   Review

3   Antepartum care   23
4   Intrapartum care   49
5   Postpartum care   73
6   Neonatal care   85

Part III   Questions & answers

7   Antepartum care   105
8   Intrapartum care   123
9   Postpartum care   141
10   Neonatal care   159

References and index

Selected references   *179*

Index   *180*

Preface

NCLEX-RN Maternal-Neonatal Nursing Made Incredibly Easy is really two books in one. The first is designed to provide you with a detailed review of essential nursing concepts, nursing diagnoses, and clinical information you need to pass the NCLEX-RN. The second provides hundreds of challenging questions, answers, and detailed rationales following the NCLEX 2010 test plan. The content review section follows the same chapter structure as the Q&A section to help you organize your study.

The content section is presented in the appealing and effective style of the *Incredibly Easy* series. Its humor encourages you to relax and have fun while learning. You will also find these valuable features in every chapter of the review:

- **Brush up on key concepts** provides an overview of anatomy and physiology.
- **Cheat sheets** provide you with a concise overview of key signs and symptoms, test results, treatments, and interventions of common diseases. Use this feature to quickly review the material you will cover in depth in the *Polish up on client care* section.
- **Keep abreast of diagnostic tests** highlights the most important tests for the disorders being discussed, including pertinent nursing actions you will need to perform to ensure client safety—a key area of NCLEX-RN testing.
- **Polish up on client care** provides a thorough review of disorders with a focus on the expected nursing care. Starting with a description of the problem, this section also covers causes, assessment findings, diagnostic test results, nursing diagnoses, treatments, and drug therapy for each disorder. Key interventions and their rationales are also provided.

In addition to your nursing knowledge, your test-taking skills can help you pass the exam. This book introduces you to the NCLEX-RN exam structure and covers techniques that will help you learn how to read test questions and understand what they are really asking—skills that are vital to NCLEX success. You also have access to study strategies, such as scheduling study time, maintaining your concentration, and finding the right study space.

Questions, Questions, and More Questions

The more you become accustomed to the styles and types of questions that may be asked, the more successful you will be on the actual exam, and that's a special strength of this book. You will find *Pump up on practice questions* at the end of each chapter, and in addition you will find an entire second section of the book featuring hundreds of additional questions. The easy-to-use format features questions on the left and answers on the right side of the same page. The questions help you assess and remember what you've just reviewed and determine areas in which you might need further review. Detailed rationales for both correct and incorrect answers are provided, and each answer provides information on the client needs category, the cognitive level of the question, and the nursing process. Helpful hints are scattered throughout the practice questions. These hints greatly increase your ability to determine the correct answer, retain important content information, and learn essential test-taking strategies. In addition, the graphics keep you focused and help build your confidence.

Be proud of your accomplishments and of your decision to prepare yourself well for the NCLEX-RN. You've worked hard to come this far. Now it's time to prepare, to practice, to build your confidence, and to succeed!

Part I   Getting ready

1   Preparing for the NCLEX®   **3**

2   Strategies for success   **15**

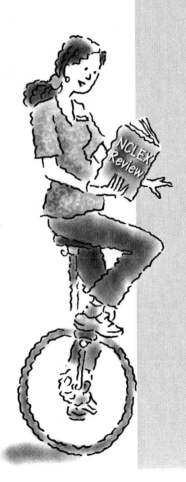

1 Preparing for the NCLEX®

In this chapter, you'll learn:

✐ why you must take the NCLEX

✐ what you need to know about taking the NCLEX by computer

✐ strategies to use when answering NCLEX questions

✐ how to recognize and answer NCLEX alternate-format questions

✐ how to avoid common mistakes when taking the NCLEX.

NCLEX basics

Passing the National Council Licensure Examination (NCLEX®) is an important landmark in your career as a nurse. The first step on your way to passing the NCLEX is to understand what it is and how it's administered.

NCLEX structure

The *NCLEX* is a test written by nurses who, like most of your nursing instructors, have an advanced degree and clinical expertise in a particular area. Only one small difference distinguishes nurses who write NCLEX questions: They're trained to write questions in a style particular to the NCLEX.

If you've completed an accredited nursing program, you've already taken numerous tests written by nurses with backgrounds and experiences similar to those of the nurses who write for the NCLEX. The test-taking experience you've already gained will help you pass the NCLEX. So your NCLEX review should be just that — a review. (For eligibility and immigration requirements for nurses from outside of the United States, see *Guidelines for international nurses,* page 4.)

What's the point of it all?
The NCLEX is designed for one purpose: namely, to determine whether it's appropriate for you to receive a license to practice as a nurse. By passing the NCLEX, you demonstrate that you possess the minimum level of knowledge necessary to practice nursing safely.

Mix 'em up
In nursing school, you probably took courses that were separated into such subjects as pharmacology, nursing leadership, health assessment, adult health, pediatric, maternal-neonatal, and psychiatric nursing. In contrast, the NCLEX is integrated, meaning that different subjects are mixed together.

As you answer NCLEX questions, you may encounter clients in any stage of life, from neonatal to geriatric. These clients — clients, in NCLEX lingo — may be of any background, may be completely well or extremely ill, and may have any disorder.

Client needs, front and center
The NCLEX draws questions from four categories of client needs that were developed by the *National Council of State Boards of Nursing* (NCSBN), the organization that sponsors and manages the NCLEX. *Client needs categories* ensure that a wide variety of topics appear on every NCLEX examination.

The NCSBN developed client needs categories after conducting a practice analysis of new nurses. All aspects of nursing care observed in the study were broken down into four main categories, some of which were broken down further into subcategories. (See *Client needs categories,* page 5.)

The whole kit and caboodle
The categories and subcategories are used to develop the *NCLEX test plan,* the content guidelines for the distribution of test questions. Question-writers and the people who put the NCLEX together use the test plan and client needs categories to make sure that a full spectrum of nursing activities is covered in the examination. Client needs categories appear in most NCLEX review and question-and-answer books, including this one. As a test-taker, you don't have to concern yourself with client needs categories. You'll see those categories for each question and answer in this book, but they'll be invisible on the actual NCLEX.

Guidelines for international nurses

To become eligible to work as a registered nurse in the United States, you'll need to complete several steps. In addition to passing the NCLEX® examination, you may need to obtain a certificate and credentials evaluation from the Commission on Graduates of Foreign Nursing Schools (CGFNS®) and acquire a visa. Requirements vary from state to state, so it's important that you first contact the Board of Nursing in the state where you want to practice nursing.

CGFNS CERTIFICATION PROGRAM

Most states require that you obtain CGFNS certification. This certification requires:
• review and authentication of your credentials, including your nursing education, registration, and licensure
• passing score on the CGFNS Qualifying Examination of nursing knowledge
• passing score on an English language proficiency test.

To be eligible to take the CGFNS Qualifying Examination, you must complete a minimum number of classroom and clinical practice hours in medical-surgical nursing, maternal-infant nursing, pediatric nursing, and psychiatric and mental health nursing from a government-approved nursing school. You must also be registered as a first-level nurse in your country of education and currently hold a license as a registered nurse in some jurisdiction.

The CGFNS Qualifying Examination is a paper and pencil test that includes 260 multiple-choice questions and is administered under controlled testing conditions. Because the test is designed to predict your likelihood of successfully passing the NCLEX-RN examination, it's based on the NCLEX-RN test plan.

You may select from three English proficiency examinations—Test of English as a Foreign Language (TOEFL®), Test of English for International Communication (TOEIC®), or International English Language Testing System (IELTS). Each test has different passing scores, and the scores are valid for up to 2 years.

CGFNS CREDENTIALS EVALUATION SERVICE

This evaluation is a comprehensive report that analyzes and compares your education and licensure with U.S. standards. It's prepared by CGFNS for a state board of nursing, an immigration office, employer, or university. To use this service you must complete an application, submit appropriate documentation, and pay a fee.

More information about the CGFNS certification program and credentials evaluation service is available at *www.cgfns.org*.

VISA REQUIRED

You can't legally immigrate to work in the United States without an occupational visa (temporary or permanent) from the United States Citizenship and Immigration Services (USCIS). The visa process is separate from the CGFNS certification process, although some of the same steps are involved. Some visas require prior CGFNS certification and a *VisaScreen*™ Certificate from the International Commission on Healthc are Professions (ICHP). The VisaScreen program involves:
• credentials review of your nursing education and current registration or licensure
• successful completion of either the CGFNS certification program or the NCLEX-RN to provide proof of nursing knowledge
• passing score on an approved English language proficiency examination.

After you successfully complete all parts of the *VisaScreen* program, you'll receive a certificate to present to the USCIS. The visa granting process can take up to one year.

You can obtain more detailed information about visa applications at *www.uscis.gov*.

Testing by computer

Like many standardized tests today, the NCLEX is administered by computer. That means you won't be filling in empty circles, sharpening pencils, or erasing frantically. It also means that you must become familiar with computer tests, if you aren't already. Fortunately, the skills required to take the NCLEX on a computer are simple enough to

Client needs categories

Each question on the NCLEX is assigned a category based on client needs. This chart lists client needs categories and subcategories and the percentages of each type of question that appears on an NCLEX examination.

Category	Subcategories	Percentage of NCLEX questions
Safe and effective care environment	• Management of care • Safety and infection control	16% to 22% 8% to 14%
Health promotion and maintenance		6% to 12%
Psychosocial integrity		6% to 12%
Physiological integrity	• Basic care and comfort • Pharmacological and parenteral therapies • Reduction of risk potential • Physiological adaptation	6% to 12% 13% to 19% 10% to 16% 11% to 17%

allow you to focus on the questions, not the keyboard.

Q&A

When you take the test, depending on the question format, you'll be presented with a question and four or more possible answers, a blank space in which to enter your answer, a figure on which you'll identify the correct area by clicking the mouse on it, a series of charts or exhibits you'll use to select the correct response, items you must rearrange in priority order by dragging and dropping them in place, an audio recording to listen to in order to select the correct response, or a question and four graphic options.

Feeling smart? Think hard!

The NCLEX is a *computer-adaptive test*, meaning that the computer reacts to the answers you give, supplying more difficult questions if you answer correctly, and slightly easier questions if you answer incorrectly. Each test is thus uniquely adapted to the individual test-taker.

A matter of time

You have a great deal of flexibility with the amount of time you can spend on individual questions. The examination lasts a maximum of 6 hours, however, so don't waste time. If you fail to answer a set number of questions within 6 hours, the computer will determine that you lack minimum competency.

Most students have plenty of time to complete the test, so take as long as you need to get the question right without wasting time. But remember to keep moving at a decent pace to help you maintain concentration.

Difficult items = Good news

If you find as you progress through the test that the questions seem to be increasingly difficult, it's a good sign. The more questions you answer correctly, the more difficult the questions become.

Some students, though, knowing that questions get progressively harder, focus on the degree of difficulty of subsequent questions to try to figure out if they're answering questions correctly. Avoid the temptation to do this, as this may get you off track.

Free at last!

The computer test finishes when one of the following events occurs:
• You demonstrate minimum competency, according to the computer program, which

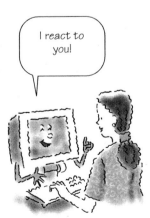

I react to you!

calculates with 95% certainty that your ability exceeds the passing standard.
• You demonstrate a lack of minimum competency, according to the computer program.
• You've answered the maximum number of questions (265 total questions).
• You've used the maximum time allowed (6 hours).

Unlocking the NCLEX mystery

In April 2004, the NCSBN added alternate-format items to the examination. However, most of the questions on the NCLEX are four-option, multiple-choice items with only one correct answer. Certain strategies can help you understand and answer any type of NCLEX question.

Alternate formats

The first type of alternate-format item is the *multiple-response question*. Unlike a traditional multiple-choice question, each multiple-response question has one or more correct answers for every question, and it may contain more than four possible answer options. You'll recognize this type of question because it will ask you to select *all* answers that apply — not just the best answer (as may be requested in the more traditional multiple-choice questions).

All or nothing
Keep in mind that, for each multiple-response question, you must select at least one answer and you must select all correct answers for the item to be counted as correct. On the NCLEX, there is no partial credit in the scoring of these items.

Don't go blank!
The second type of alternate-format item is the *fill-in-the-blank* question. These questions require you to provide the answer yourself, rather than select it from a list of options. You will perform a calculation and then type your

answer (a number, without any words, units of measurements, commas, or spaces) in the blank space provided after the question. Rules for rounding are included in the question stem if appropriate. A calculator button is provided so you can do your calculations electronically.

Mouse marks the spot!
The third type of alternate-format item is a question that asks you to identify an area on an illustration or graphic. For these *"hot spot" questions*, the computerized exam will ask you to place your cursor and click over the correct area on an illustration. Try to be as precise as possible when marking the location. As with the fill-in-the-blanks, the identification questions on the computerized exam may require extremely precise answers in order for them to be considered correct.

Click, choose, and prioritize
The fourth alternate-format item type is the *chart/exhibit* format. For this question type, you'll be given a problem and then a series of small screens with additional information you'll need to answer the question. By clicking on the tabs on screen, you can access each chart or exhibit item. After viewing the chart or exhibit, you select your answer from four multiple-choice options.

Drag n' drop
The fifth alternate-format item type involves prioritizing actions or placing a series of statements in correct order using a *drag-and-drop* (ordered response) technique. To move an answer option from the list of unordered options into the correct sequence, click on it using the mouse. While still holding down the mouse button, drag the option to the ordered response part of the screen. Release the mouse button to "drop" the option into place. Repeat this process until you've moved all of the available options into the correct order.

Now hear this!
The sixth alternate-format item type is the *audio item* format. You'll be given a set of headphones and you'll be asked to listen to an

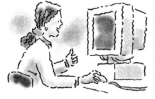

The harder it gets, the better I'm doing.

audio clip and select the correct answer from four options. You'll need to select the correct answer on the computer screen as you would with the traditional multiple-choice questions.

Picture perfect

The final alternate-format item type is the *graphic option* question. This varies from the exhibit format type because in the graphic option, your answer choices will be graphics such as ECG strips. You'll have to select the appropriate graphic to answer the question presented.

The standard's still the standard

The NCSBN hasn't yet established a percentage of alternate-format items to be administered to each candidate. In fact, your exam may contain only one alternate-format item. So relax; the standard, four-option, multiple-choice format questions constitute the bulk of the test. (See *Sample NCLEX questions*, pages 8 to 10.)

Understanding the question

NCLEX questions are commonly long. As a result, it's easy to become overloaded with information. To focus on the question and avoid becoming overwhelmed, apply proven strategies for answering NCLEX questions, including:
- determining what the question is asking
- determining relevant facts about the client
- rephrasing the question in your mind
- choosing the best option or options before entering your answer.

DETERMINE WHAT THE QUESTION IS ASKING

Read the question twice. If the answer isn't apparent, rephrase the question in simpler, more personal terms. Breaking down the question into easier, less intimidating terms may help you to focus more accurately on the correct answer.

Give it a try

For example, a question might be, "A 74-year-old client with a history of heart failure is admitted to the coronary care unit with

pulmonary edema. He's intubated and placed on a mechanical ventilator. Which parameters should the nurse monitor closely to assess the client's response to a bolus dose of furosemide (Lasix) I.V.?"

The options for this question — numbered from 1 to 4 — might include:
1. Daily weight
2. 24-hour intake and output
3. Serum sodium levels
4. Hourly urine output

Hocus, focus on the question

Read the question again, ignoring all details except what's being asked. Focus on the last line of the question. It asks you to select the appropriate assessment for monitoring a client who received a bolus of furosemide I.V.

DETERMINE WHAT FACTS ABOUT THE CLIENT ARE RELEVANT

Next, sort out the relevant client information. Start by asking whether any of the information provided about the client isn't relevant. For instance, do you need to know that the client has been admitted to the coronary care unit? Probably not; his reaction to I.V. furosemide won't be affected by his location in the hospital.

Determine what you do know about the client. In the example, you know that:
- he just received an I.V. bolus of furosemide, a crucial fact
- he has pulmonary edema, the most fundamental aspect of the client's underlying condition
- he's intubated and placed on a mechanical ventilator, suggesting that his pulmonary edema is serious
- he's 74 years old and has a history of heart failure, a fact that may or may not be relevant.

REPHRASE THE QUESTION

After you've determined relevant information about the client and the question being asked, consider rephrasing the question to make it more clear. Eliminate jargon and put the question in simpler, more personal terms. Here's how you might rephrase the question in the example: "My client has pulmonary edema. He requires intubation and

(Text continues on page 10.)

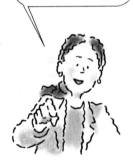

Focusing on what the question is really asking can help you choose the correct answer.

Sample NCLEX questions

Sometimes, getting used to the format is as important as knowing the material. Try your hand at these sample questions and you'll have a leg up when you take the real test!

Sample four-option, multiple-choice question

A client's arterial blood gas (ABG) results are as follows: pH, 7.16; $Paco_2$, 80 mm Hg; Pao_2, 46 mm Hg; HCO_3^-, 24 mEq/L; Sao_2, 81%. These ABG results represent which condition?

1. Metabolic acidosis
2. Metabolic alkalosis
3. Respiratory acidosis
4. Respiratory alkalosis

Correct answer: 3

Sample multiple-response question

A nurse is caring for a 45-year-old married woman who has undergone hemicolectomy for colon cancer. The woman has two children. Which concepts about families should the nurse keep in mind when providing care for this client?

Select all that apply:
1. Illness in one family member can affect all members.
2. Family roles don't change because of illness.
3. A family member may have more than one role at a time in the family.
4. Children typically aren't affected by adult illness.
5. The effects of an illness on a family depend on the stage of the family's life cycle.
6. Changes in sleeping and eating patterns may be signs of stress in a family.

Correct answer: 1, 3, 5, 6

Sample fill-in-the-blank calculation question

An infant who weighs 8 kg is to receive ampicillin 25 mg/kg I.V. every 6 hours. How many milligrams should the nurse administer per dose? Record your answer using a whole number.

_____ milligrams

Correct answer: 200

Sample hot spot question

A client has a history of aortic stenosis. Identify the area where the nurse should place the stethoscope to best hear the murmur.

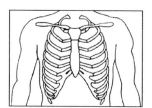

Correct answer:

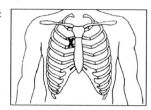

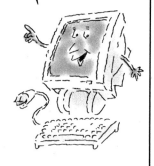

I can be ambivalent. More than one answer may be correct.

Sample NCLEX questions *(continued)*

Sample exhibit question

A 3-year old child is being treated for severe status asthmaticus. After reviewing the progress notes (shown below), the nurse should determine that this client is being treated for which condition?

Progress notes	
9/1/10 0600	Pt. was acutely restless, diaphoretic, and with dyspnea at 0530. Dr. T. Smith notified of findings at 0545 and ordered ABG analysis. ABG drawn from R radial artery. Stat results as follows: pH 7.28, Paco$_2$ SS mm Hg, HCO$_3$- 26 mEg/L. Dr. Smith with pt. now. _____ J. Collins, RN.

1. Metabolic acidosis
2. Respiratory alkalosis
3. Respiratory acidosis
4. Metabolic alkalosis

Correct answer: 3

Sample drag-and-drop (ordered response) question

When teaching an antepartal client about the passage of the fetus through the birth canal during labor, the nurse describes the cardinal mechanisms of labor. Place these events in the sequence in which they occur. Use all options:

1. Flexion	
2. External rotation	
3. Descent	
4. Expulsion	
5. Internal rotation	
6. Extension	

Correct answer:

3. Descent
1. Flexion
5. Internal rotation
6. Extension
2. External rotation
4. Expulsion

(continued)

Sample NCLEX questions *(continued)*

Sample audio item question

Listen to the audio clip. What sound do you hear in the bases of this client with heart failure?

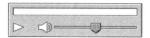

1. Crackles
2. Rhonchi
3. Wheezes
4. Pleural friction rub

Correct answer: 1

Sample graphic option question

Which electrocardiogram strip should the nurse document as sinus tachycardia?

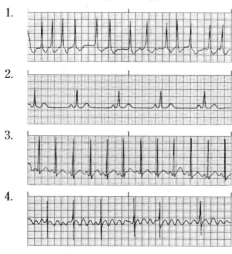

Correct answer: 1

---

mechanical ventilation. He's 74 years old and has a history of heart failure. He received an I.V. bolus of furosemide. What assessment parameter should I monitor?"

CHOOSE THE BEST OPTION

Armed with all the information you now have, it's time to select an option. You know that the client received an I.V. bolus of furosemide, a diuretic. You know that monitoring fluid intake and output is a key nursing intervention for a client taking a diuretic, a fact that eliminates options 1 and 3 (daily weight and serum sodium levels), narrowing the answer down to option 2 or 4 (24-hour intake and output or hourly urine output).

Can I use a lifeline?

You also know that the drug was administered by I.V. bolus, suggesting a rapid effect. (In fact, furosemide administered by I.V. bolus takes effect almost immediately.)

Monitoring the client's 24-hour intake and output would be appropriate for assessing the effects of repeated doses of furosemide. Hourly urine output, however, is most appropriate in this situation because it monitors the immediate effect of this rapid-acting drug.

Key strategies

Regardless of the type of question, four key strategies will help you determine the correct answer for each question. These strategies are:
- considering the nursing process
- referring to Maslow's hierarchy of needs
- reviewing client safety
- reflecting on principles of therapeutic communication.

Nursing process

One of the ways to answer a question is to apply the nursing process. Steps in the nursing process include:
- assessment
- diagnosis
- planning
- implementation
- evaluation.

First things first
The nursing process may provide insights that help you analyze a question. According to the nursing process, assessment comes before analysis, which comes before planning, which comes before implementation, which comes before evaluation.

You're halfway to the correct answer when you encounter a four-option, multiple-choice question that asks you to assess the situation and then provides two assessment options and two implementation options. You can immediately eliminate the implementation options, which then gives you, at worst, a 50-50 chance of selecting the correct answer. Use the following sample question to apply the nursing process:

A client returns from an endoscopic procedure during which he was sedated.

Before offering the client food, which action should the nurse take?
1. Assess the client's respiratory status.
2. Check the client's gag reflex.
3. Place the client in a side-lying position.
4. Have the client drink a few sips of water.

Assess before intervening
According to the nursing process, the nurse must assess a client before performing an intervention. Does the question indicate that the client has been properly assessed? No, it doesn't. Therefore, you can eliminate options 3 and 4 because they're both interventions.

That leaves options 1 and 2, both of which are assessments. Your nursing knowledge should tell you the correct answer — in this case, option 2. The sedation required for an endoscopic procedure may impair the client's gag reflex, so you would assess the gag reflex before giving food to the client to reduce the risk of aspiration and airway obstruction.

Final elimination
Why not select option 1, assessing the client's respiratory status? You might select this option but the question is specifically asking about offering the client food, an action that wouldn't be taken if the client's respiratory status was at all compromised. In this case, you're making a judgment based on the phrase, "Before offering the client food." If the question was trying to test your knowledge of respiratory depression following an endoscopic procedure, it probably wouldn't mention a function — such as giving food to a client — that clearly occurs only after the client's respiratory status has been stabilized.

Maslow's hierarchy

Knowledge of Maslow's hierarchy of needs can be a vital tool for establishing priorities on the NCLEX. Maslow's theory states that physiologic needs are the most basic human needs of all. Only after physiologic needs have been met can safety concerns be addressed. Only after safety concerns are met can concerns involving love and belonging be addressed, and so forth. Apply the principles of Maslow's hierarchy of needs to the following sample question:

A client complains of severe pain 2 days after surgery. Which action should the nurse perform first?

1. Offer reassurance to the client that he will feel less pain tomorrow.
2. Allow the client time to verbalize his feelings.
3. Check the client's vital signs.
4. Administer an analgesic.

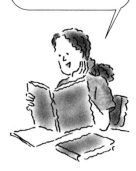

Say it 1,000 times: Studying for the exam is fun... studying for the exam is fun...

Phys before psych
In this example, two of the options — 3 and 4 — address physiologic needs. Options 1 and 2 address psychosocial concerns. According to Maslow, physiologic needs must be met before psychosocial needs, so you can eliminate options 1 and 2.

Final elimination
Now, use your nursing knowledge to choose the best answer from the two remaining options. In this case, option 3 is correct because the client's vital signs should be checked before administering an analgesic (assessment before intervention). When prioritizing according to Maslow's hierarchy, remember your ABCs — airway, breathing, circulation — to help you further prioritize. Check for a patent airway before addressing breathing. Check breathing before checking the health of the cardiovascular system.

One caveat...
Just because an option appears on the NCLEX doesn't mean it's a viable choice for the client referred to in the question. Always examine your choice in light of your knowledge and experience. Ask yourself, "Does this choice make sense for this client?" Allow yourself to eliminate choices — even ones that might normally take priority — if they don't make sense for a particular client's situation.

Client safety

As you might expect, client safety takes high priority on the NCLEX. You'll encounter

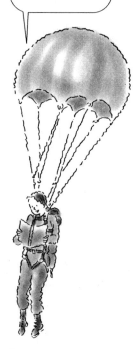

Client safety takes a high priority on the NCLEX.

many questions that can be answered by asking yourself, "Which answer will best ensure the safety of this client?" Use client safety criteria for situations involving laboratory values, drug administration, activities of daily living, or nursing care procedures.

Client first, equipment second
You may encounter a question in which some options address the client and others address the equipment. When in doubt, select an option relating to the client; never place equipment before a client.

For example, suppose a question asks what the nurse should do first when entering a client's room where an infusion pump alarm is sounding. If two options deal with the infusion pump, one with the infusion tubing, and another with the client's catheter insertion site, select the one relating to the client's catheter insertion site. Always check the client first; the equipment can wait.

Therapeutic communication

Some NCLEX questions focus on the nurse's ability to communicate effectively with the client. Therapeutic communication incorporates verbal or nonverbal responses and involves:
- listening to the client
- understanding the client's needs
- promoting clarification and insight about the client's condition.

Room for improvement
Like other NCLEX questions, those dealing with therapeutic communication commonly require choosing the best response. First, eliminate options that indicate the use of poor therapeutic communication techniques, such as those in which the nurse:
- tells the client what to do without regard to the client's feelings or desires (the "do this" response)
- asks a question that can be answered "yes" or "no," or with another one-syllable response
- seeks reasons for the client's behavior
- implies disapproval of the client's behavior
- offers false reassurances

- attempts to interpret the client's behavior rather than allow the client to verbalize his own feelings
- offers a response that focuses on the nurse, not the client.

Ah, that's better!

When answering NCLEX questions, look for responses that:
- allow the client time to think and reflect
- encourage the client to talk
- encourage the client to describe a particular experience
- reflect that the nurse has listened to the client, such as through paraphrasing the client's response.

Avoiding pitfalls

Even the most knowledgeable students can get tripped up on certain NCLEX questions. (See *A tricky question*, page 14.) Students commonly cite three areas that can be difficult for unwary test-takers:

 knowing the difference between the NCLEX and the "real world"

delegating care

knowing laboratory values.

NCLEX versus the real world

Some students who take the NCLEX have extensive practical experience in health care. For example, many test-takers have worked as licensed practical nurses or nursing assistants. In one of those capacities, test-takers might have been exposed to less than optimum clinical practice and may carry those experiences over to the NCLEX.

However, the NCLEX is a textbook examination — not a test of clinical skills. Take the NCLEX with the understanding that what happens in the real world may differ from what the NCLEX and your nursing school say should happen.

Don't take shortcuts

If you've had practical experience in health care, you may know a quicker way to perform a procedure or tricks to get by when you don't have the right equipment. Situations such as staff shortages may force you to improvise. On the NCLEX, such scenarios can lead to trouble. Always check your practical experiences against textbook nursing care, taking care to select the response that follows the textbook.

Delegating care

On the NCLEX, you may encounter questions that assess your ability to delegate care. Delegating care involves coordinating the efforts of other health care workers to provide effective care for your client. On the NCLEX, you may be asked to assign duties to:
- licensed practical nurses or licensed vocational nurses
- direct-care workers, such as certified nursing assistants and personal care aides
- other support staff, such as nutrition assistants and housekeepers.

In addition, you'll be asked to decide when to notify a physician, a social worker, or another hospital staff member. In each case, you'll have to decide when, where, and how to delegate.

Shoulds and shouldn'ts

As a general rule, it's okay to delegate actions that involve stable clients or standard, unchanging procedures. Bathing, feeding, dressing, and transferring clients are examples of procedures that can be delegated.

Be careful not to delegate complicated or complex activities. In addition, don't delegate activities that involve assessment, evaluation, or your own nursing judgment. On the NCLEX and in the real world, these duties fall squarely on your shoulders. Make sure that you take primary responsibility for assessing and evaluating the client and for making decisions about the client's care. Never hand off those responsibilities to someone with less training.

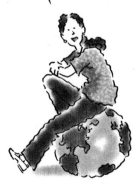

Remember, this is an exam, not the real world.

Normal laboratory values

- Blood urea nitrogen: 8 to 25 mg/dl
- Creatinine: 0.6 to 1.5 mg/dl
- Sodium: 135 to 145 mmol/L
- Potassium: 3.5 to 5.5 mEq/L
- Chloride: 97 to 110 mmol/L
- Glucose (fasting plasma): 70 to 110 mg/dl
- Hemoglobin
  Male: 13.8 to 17.2 g/dl
  Female: 12.1 to 15.1 g/dl
- Hematocrit
  Male: 40.7% to 50.3%
  Female: 36.1% to 44.3%

Advice from the experts

A tricky question

The NCLEX occasionally asks a particular kind of question called the "further teaching" question, which involves client-teaching situations. These questions can be tricky. You'll have to choose the response that suggests the client has *not* learned the correct information. Here's an example:

37. A client undergoes a total hip replacement. Which statement by the client indicates he requires further teaching?
1. "I'll need to keep several pillows between my legs at night."
2. "I'll need to remember not to cross my legs. It's such a bad habit."
3. "The occupational therapist is showing me how to use a 'sock puller' to help me get dressed."
4. "I don't know if I'll be able to get off that low toilet seat at home by myself."

The option you should choose here is 4 because it indicates that the client has a poor understanding of the precautions required after a total hip replacement and that he needs further teaching. Remember: If you see the phrase further teaching or further instruction, you're looking for a wrong answer by the client.

Calling in reinforcements

Deciding when to notify a physician, a social worker, or another hospital staff member is an important element of nursing care. On the NCLEX, however, choices that involve notifying the physician are usually incorrect. Remember that the NCLEX wants to see you, the nurse, at work.

If you're sure the correct answer is to notify the physician, though, make sure the client's safety has been addressed before notifying a physician or another staff member. On the NCLEX, the client's safety has a higher priority than notifying other health care providers.

Knowing laboratory values

Some NCLEX questions supply laboratory results without indicating normal levels. As a result, answering questions involving laboratory values requires you to have the normal range of the most common laboratory values memorized to make an informed decision (See *Normal laboratory values.*)

2 Strategies for success

In this chapter, you'll review:

✐ how to properly prepare for the NCLEX

✐ how to concentrate during difficult study times

✐ how to make more effective use of your time

✐ how creative studying strategies can enhance learning.

Study preparations

If you're like most people preparing to take the NCLEX®, you're probably feeling nervous, anxious, or concerned. Keep in mind that most test takers pass the first time around.

Passing the test won't happen by accident, though; you'll need to prepare carefully and efficiently. To help jump-start your preparations:
- determine your strengths and weaknesses
- create a study schedule
- set realistic goals
- find an effective study space
- think positively
- start studying sooner rather than later.

Strengths and weaknesses

Most students recognize that, even at the end of their nursing studies, they know more about some topics than others. Because the NCLEX covers a broad range of material, you should make some decisions about how intensively you'll review each topic.

Make a list
Base those decisions on a list. Divide a sheet of paper in half vertically. On one side, list topics you think you know well. On the other side, list topics you feel less secure about. Pay no attention if one side is longer than the other. When you're done studying, you'll feel strong in every area.

Where the list comes from
To make sure your list reflects a comprehensive view of all the areas you studied in school, look at the contents page in the front of this book. For each topic listed, place it in the "know well" column or "needs review"

column. Separating content areas this way shows immediately which topics need less study time and which need more time.

Scheduling study time

Study when you're most alert. Most people can identify a period of the day when they feel most alert. If you feel most alert and energized in the morning, for example, set aside sections of time in the morning for topics that need a lot of review. Then you can use the evening to study topics for which you just need some refreshing. The opposite is true as well; if you're more alert in the evening, study difficult topics at that time.

What you'll do, when
Set up a basic schedule for studying. Using a calendar or organizer, determine how much time remains before you'll take the NCLEX. (See *2 to 3 months before the NCLEX,* page 16.) Fill in the remaining days with specific times and topics to be studied. For example, you might schedule the respiratory system on a Tuesday morning and the GI system that afternoon. Remember to schedule difficult topics during your most alert times.

Keep in mind that you shouldn't fill each day with studying. Be realistic and set aside time for normal activities. Try to create ample study time before the NCLEX and then stick to the schedule. Allow some extra time in the schedule in case you get behind or come across a topic that requires extra review.

Set goals you can meet
Part of creating a schedule means setting goals you can accomplish. You no doubt studied a great deal in nursing school, and by now you have a sense of your own capabilities. Ask yourself, "How much can I cover in a day?" Set that amount of time aside and

To-do list

2 to 3 months before the NCLEX

With 2 to 3 months remaining before you plan to take the examination, take these steps:
• Establish a study schedule. Set aside ample time to study but also leave time for social activities, exercise, family or personal responsibilities, and other matters.
• Become knowledgeable about the NCLEX-RN, its content, the types of questions it asks, and the testing format.
• Begin studying your notes, texts, and other study materials.
• Answer some NCLEX practice questions to help you diagnose strengths and weaknesses as well as to become familiar with NCLEX-style questions.

then stay on task. You'll feel better about yourself — and your chances of passing the NCLEX — when you meet your goals regularly.

Study space

Find a space conducive to effective learning and then study there. Whatever you do, don't study with a television on in the room. Instead, find a quiet, inviting study space that:
• is located in a quiet, convenient place, away from normal traffic patterns
• contains a solid chair that encourages good posture (Avoid studying in bed; you'll be more likely to fall asleep and not accomplish your goals.)
• uses comfortable, soft lighting with which you can see clearly without eye strain
• has a temperature between 65° and 70° F
• contains flowers or green plants, familiar photos or paintings, and easy access to soft, instrumental background music.

Accentuate the positive
Consider taping positive messages around your study space. Make signs with words of encouragement, such as, "You can do it!" "Keep studying!" and "Remember the goal!" These upbeat messages can help keep you going when your attention begins to waver.

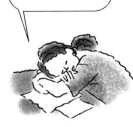

Approach your studying with enthusiasm, sincerity, and determination.

Maintaining concentration

When you're faced with reviewing the amount of information covered by the NCLEX, it's easy to become distracted and lose your concentration. When you lose concentration, you make less effective use of valuable study time. To stay focused, keep these tips in mind:
• Alternate the order of the subjects you study during the day to add variety to your study. Try alternating between topics you find most interesting and those you find least interesting.
• Approach your studying with enthusiasm, sincerity, and determination.
• Once you've decided to study, begin immediately. Don't let anything interfere with your thought processes once you've begun.
• Concentrate on accomplishing one task at a time, to the exclusion of everything else.
• Don't try to do two things at once, such as studying and watching television or conversing with friends.
• Work continuously without interruption for a while, but don't study for such a long period that the whole experience becomes grueling or boring.
• Allow time for periodic breaks to give yourself a change of pace. Use these breaks to ease your transition into studying a new topic.

• When studying in the evening, wind down from your studies slowly. Don't progress directly from studying to sleeping.

Taking care of yourself

Never neglect your physical and mental well-being in favor of longer study hours. Maintaining physical and mental health are critical for success in taking the NCLEX. (See *4 to 6 weeks before the NCLEX*.)

A few simple rules
You can increase your likelihood of passing the test by following these simple health rules:
• Get plenty of rest. You can't think deeply or concentrate for long periods when you're tired.
• Eat nutritious meals. Maintaining your energy level is impossible when you're undernourished.
• Exercise regularly. Regular exercise, preferably 30 minutes daily, helps you work harder and think more clearly. As a result, you'll study more efficiently and increase the likelihood of success on the all-important NCLEX.

Memory powers, activate!
If you're having trouble concentrating but would rather push through than take a break, try making your studying more active by reading out loud. Active studying can renew

your powers of concentration. By reading review material out loud to yourself, you're engaging your ears as well as your eyes — and making your studying a more active process. Hearing the material out loud also fosters memory and subsequent recall.

You can also rewrite in your own words a few of the more difficult concepts you're reviewing. Explaining these concepts in writing forces you to think through the material and can jump-start your memory.

Study schedule

When you were creating your schedule, you might have asked yourself, "How long should I study? One hour at a stretch? Two hours? Three?" To make the best use of your study time, you'll need to answer those questions.

Optimum study time

Consider studying in 20- to 30-minute intervals with a short break in-between. You remember the material you study at the beginning and end of a session best and tend to remember less material studied in the middle of the session. The total length of time in each study session depends on you and the amount of material you need to cover.

> Kowabonga! Regular exercise helps you work harder and think more clearly.

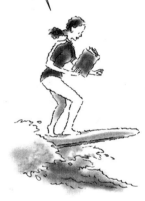

To-do list

4 to 6 weeks before the NCLEX

With 4 to 6 weeks remaining before you plan to take the examination, take these steps:
• Focus on your areas of weakness. That way, you'll have time to review these areas again before the test date.
• Find a study partner or form a study group.
• Take a practice test to gauge your skill level early.
• Take time to eat, sleep, exercise, and socialize to avoid burnout.

To-do list

1 week before the NCLEX

With 1 week remaining before the NCLEX examination, take these steps:
- Take a review test to measure your progress.
- Record key ideas and principles on note cards or audiotapes.
- Rest, eat well, and avoid thinking about the examination during nonstudy times.
- Treat yourself to one special event. You've been working hard, and you deserve it!

To thine own self be true

So what's the answer? It doesn't matter as long as you determine what's best for you. At the beginning of your NCLEX study schedule, try study periods of varying lengths. Pay close attention to those that seem more successful.

Remember that you're a trained nurse who is competent at assessment. Think of yourself as a client, and assess your own progress. Then implement the strategy that works best for you.

Finding time to study

So does that mean that short sections of time are useless? Not at all. We all have spaces in our day that might otherwise be dead time. (See *1 week before the NCLEX*.) These are perfect times to review for the NCLEX but not to cover new material because, by the time you get deep into new material, your time will be over. Always keep some flash cards or a small notebook handy for situations when you have a few extra minutes.

You'll be amazed how many short sessions you can find in a day and how much reviewing you can do in 5 minutes. The following occasions offer short stretches of time you can use for studying:
- eating breakfast
- waiting for, or riding on, a train or bus
- waiting in line at the bank, post office, bookstore, or other places
- using exercise equipment, such as a treadmill.

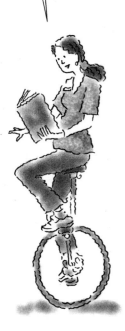

Studying getting dull? Get creative and liven it up.

Creative studying

Even when you study in a perfect study space and concentrate better than ever, studying for the NCLEX can get a little, well, dull. Even people with terrific study habits occasionally feel bored or sluggish. That's why it's important to have some creative tricks in your study bag to liven up your studying during those down times.

Creative studying doesn't have to be hard work. It involves making efforts to alter your study habits a bit. Some techniques that might help include studying with a partner or group and creating flash cards or other audio-visual study tools.

Study partners

Studying with a partner or group of students (3 or 4 students at most) can be an excellent way to energize your studying. Working with a partner allows you to test each other on the material you've reviewed. Your partner can give you encouragement and motivation. Perhaps most important, working with a partner can provide a welcome break from solitary studying.

What to look for in a partner

Exercise some care when choosing a study partner or assembling a study group. A partner who doesn't fit your needs won't help you make the most of your study time. Look for a partner who:

• possesses similar goals to yours. For example, someone taking the NCLEX at approximately the same date who feels the same sense of urgency as you do might make an excellent partner.

• possesses about the same level of knowledge as you. Tutoring someone can sometimes help you learn, but partnering should be give-and-take so both partners can gain knowledge.

• can study without excess chatting or interruptions. Socializing is an important part of creative study but, remember, you still have to pass the NCLEX — so stay serious!

Audiovisual tools

Using flash cards and other audiovisual tools fosters retention and makes learning and reviewing fun.

Flash Gordon? No, it's Flash Card!

Flash cards can provide you with an excellent study tool. The process of writing material on a flash card will help you remember it. In addition, flash cards are small and easily portable, perfect for those 5-minute slivers of time that show up during the day.

Creating a flash card should be fun. Use magic markers, highlighters, and other colorful tools to make them visually stimulating. The more effort you put into creating your flash cards, the better you'll remember the material contained on the cards.

Other visual tools

Flowcharts, drawings, diagrams, and other image-oriented study aids can also help you learn material more effectively. Substituting images for text can be a great way to give your eyes a break and recharge your brain. Remember to use vivid colors to make your creations visually engaging.

Hear's the thing

If you learn more effectively when you hear information rather than see it, consider recording key ideas using a handheld tape recorder. Recording information helps promote memory because you say the information aloud when taping and then listen to it when playing it back. Like flash cards, tapes are portable and perfect for those short study periods during the day. (See *The day before the NCLEX*.)

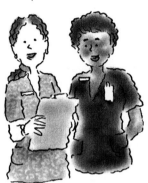

It wasn't easy finding a partner who has the same study habits I do.

To-do list

The day before the NCLEX

With 1 day before the NCLEX examination, take these steps:

• Drive to the test site, review traffic patterns, and find out where to park. If your route to the test site occurs during heavy traffic or if you're expecting bad weather, set aside extra time to ensure prompt arrival.

• Do something relaxing during the day.

• Avoid concentrating on the test.

• Eat well and avoid dwelling on the NCLEX during nonstudy periods.

• Call a supportive friend or relative for some last-minute words of encouragement.

• Get plenty of rest the night before and allow plenty of time in the morning.

To-do list

The day of the NCLEX

On the day of the NCLEX examination, take these steps:
• Get up early.
• Wear comfortable clothes, preferably with layers you can adjust to fit the room temperature.
• Leave your house early.
• Arrive at the test site early with required paperwork in hand.
• Avoid looking at your notes as you wait for your test computer.
• Listen carefully to the instructions given before entering the test room.

Good luck!

> Practice questions provide an excellent means of marking your progress.

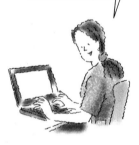

Practice questions

Practice questions should be an important part of your NCLEX study strategy. Practice questions can improve your studying by helping you review material and familiarizing yourself with the exact style of questions you'll encounter on the NCLEX.

Practice at the beginning
Consider working through some practice questions as soon as you begin studying for the NCLEX. For example, you might try a few of the questions that appear at the end of each chapter in this book.

If you do well, you probably know the material contained in that chapter fairly well and can spend less time reviewing that particular topic. If you have trouble with the questions, spend extra study time on that topic.

I'm getting there
Practice questions can also provide an excellent means of marking your progress. Don't worry if you have trouble answering the first few practice questions you take; you'll need time to adjust to the way the questions are asked. Eventually you'll become accustomed to the question format and begin to focus more on the questions themselves.

If you make practice questions a regular part of your study regimen, you'll be able to notice areas in which you're improving. You can then adjust your study time accordingly.

Practice makes perfect
As you near the examination date, you should increase the number of NCLEX practice questions you answer at one sitting. This will enable you to approximate the experience of taking the actual NCLEX examination. Note that 75 questions is the minimum number of questions you'll be asked on the actual NCLEX examination. By gradually tackling larger practice tests, you'll increase your confidence, build test-taking endurance, and strengthen the concentration skills that enable you to succeed on the NCLEX. (See *The day of the NCLEX*.)

Part II   Review

3   Antepartum care   23

4   Intrapartum care   49

5   Postpartum care   73

6   Neonatal care   85

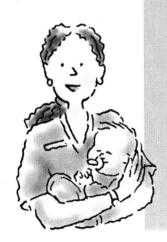

3 Antepartum care

In this chapter, you'll review:

✐ basics of antepartum care

✐ antepartum tests and procedures

✐ common antepartum disorders and complications.

Brush up on key concepts

Antepartum care refers to care of a mother before childbirth. Knowledge of the physiologic changes that accompany pregnancy and fetal development is essential to understanding client care during the antepartum period.

At any time, you can review the major points of this chapter by consulting the *Cheat sheet* on pages 24 to 26.

Normal antepartum period

Nursing care during the normal antepartum period includes taking a thorough maternal history, performing a complete physical examination, and educating the client about antepartum health.

SIGNS AND SYMPTOMS OF PREGNANCY

The client may experience presumptive, probable, or positive signs of pregnancy.

Could be

Presumptive signs of pregnancy include:
• amenorrhea or slight, painless spotting of unknown cause in early gestation
• breast enlargement and tenderness
• fatigue
• increased skin pigmentation
• nausea and vomiting
• quickening (first recognizable movement of fetus)
• urinary frequency and urgency.

Probably is

Probable signs of pregnancy include:
• ballottement (passive fetal movement in response to tapping the lower portion of the uterus or cervix)
• Braxton Hicks contractions (painless uterine contractions that occur throughout pregnancy)
• Chadwick's sign (color of the vaginal walls changes from normal light pink to deep violet)
• Goodell's sign (softening of the cervix)
• Hegar's sign (softening of the lower uterine segment) may be present at 6 to 8 weeks' gestation
• positive pregnancy test results
• abdominal and uterine enlargement
• abdominal strain.

Definitely is

Positive signs of pregnancy include:
• detection of fetal heartbeat (by 17 to 20 weeks' gestation)
• detection of fetal movements (after 16 weeks' gestation)
• ultrasound findings (as early as 6 weeks' gestation).

PHYSIOLOGIC ADAPTATIONS

Here's a review of how body systems adapt to pregnancy.

My ever changin' heart

Cardiovascular system changes include:
• cardiac hypertrophy from increased blood volume and cardiac output
• displacement of the heart upward and to the left from pressure on the diaphragm
• progressive increase in blood volume, peaking in the third trimester at 30% to 50% of levels before pregnancy
• resting pulse rate fluctuations, with increases ranging from 15 to 20 beats/minute at term

(Text continues on page 26.)

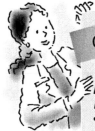

Cheat sheet

Antepartum care refresher

ACQUIRED IMMUNODEFICIENCY SYNDROME

Key signs and symptoms
- Diarrhea
- Fatigue
- Kaposi's sarcoma
- Mild flulike symptoms
- Opportunistic infections, such as toxoplasmosis, oral and vaginal candidiasis, herpes simplex, *Pneumocystis carinii*, and *Candida* esophagitis
- Anorexia and weight loss

Key test results
- CD4$^+$ T-cell level is less than 200 cells/μl.
- Enzyme-linked immunosorbent assay shows positive human immunodeficiency virus antibody titer.
- Western blot test is positive.

Key treatments
- If the client is newly diagnosed, zidovudine (Retrovir) or didanosine (Videx) treatment initiated at 14 to 34 weeks' gestation

Key interventions
- Assess whether the client can care for her infant after delivery.

ADOLESCENT PREGNANCY

Key signs and symptoms
- Denial of pregnancy, which may deter the adolescent from seeking medical attention early in the pregnancy

Key test results
- Pregnancy test is positive.

Key treatments
- Diet with caloric intake that supports the growing adolescent and her developing fetus

Key interventions
- Monitor the adolescent's weight gain.
- Advise the adolescent of her options, including terminating the pregnancy, continuing the pregnancy and giving up the infant for adoption, or continuing the pregnancy and keeping the infant.

DIABETES MELLITUS

Key signs and symptoms
- Glycosuria
- Ketonuria
- Polyuria

Key test results
- One-hour glucose tolerance test reveals glucose level greater than 140 mg/dl.

Key treatments
- 1,800- to 2,200-calorie diet divided into three meals and three snacks that should also include low fat and cholesterol and high fiber
- Insulin or glyburide (DiaBeta) after the first trimester

Key interventions
- Encourage adherence to dietary regulations.
- Encourage the client to exercise moderately.
- Prepare the client for antepartum fetal surveillance testing, including oxytocin challenge testing, nipple stimulation stress testing, amniotic fluid index, biophysical profile, and nonstress test (NST).

ECTOPIC PREGNANCY

Key signs and symptoms
- Irregular vaginal bleeding; possible amenorrhea followed by bleeding
- Abdominal or pelvic pain; may be sharp or dull
- Rupture of tubes, causing sudden and severe abdominal pain, syncope, and referred shoulder pain as the abdomen fills with blood
- Uterine size smaller than expected for gestational age

Key test results
- Human chorionic gonadotropin (HCG) titers are abnormally low when compared to a normal pregnancy.
- Serum progesterone levels are lower than in a normal pregnancy.

Key treatments
- Laparotomy to ligate the bleeding vessels and remove or repair damaged fallopian tube
- If the tube hasn't ruptured, methotrexate (Trexall) followed by leucovorin to stop trophoblastic cells from growing (therapy continues until negative HCG levels are achieved)

Key interventions
- Monitor for severe abdominal pain, orthostatic hypotension, tachycardia, and dizziness.
- Administer blood products and monitor closely during infusion.
- Administer Rh$_o$(D) immune globulin (RhoGAM) to clients who are Rh-negative.

Don't forget, pregnancy itself is NOT a disorder. Effective nursing care usually involves listening to and reassuring healthy mothers.

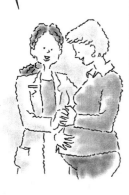

Antepartum care refresher (continued)

HEART DISEASE
Key signs and symptoms
- Tachycardia
- Dyspnea
- Fatigue
- Diastolic murmur at the heart's apex
- Crackles at the base of the lungs

Key test results
- Echocardiography, electrocardiography, and chest X-ray may reveal cardiac abnormalities, impaired cardiac function, and cardiovascular decompensation.

Key treatments
Class III and IV
- Anticoagulant: heparin
- Antiarrhythmics: digoxin (Lanoxin), procainamide, beta-adrenergic blockers
- Thiazide diuretics and furosemide (Lasix) to control heart failure if activity restriction and reduced sodium intake don't prevent it

Key interventions
- Assess cardiovascular and respiratory status.
- Administer oxygen by nasal cannula or face mask during labor.
- Position the client on her left side with her head and shoulders elevated during labor.

HYDATIDIFORM MOLE
Key signs and symptoms
- Intermittent or continuous bright red or brownish vaginal bleeding by 12 weeks' gestation
- Absence of fetal heart sounds

Key test results
- HCG levels are extremely high for early pregnancy
- Ultrasound fails to reveal a fetal skeleton.

Key treatments
- Therapeutic abortion (suction and curettage) if a spontaneous abortion doesn't occur
- Weekly monitoring of HCG levels until they remain normal for 3 consecutive weeks
- Periodic follow-up for 1 to 2 years because of increased risk of neoplasm

Key interventions
- Monitor vaginal bleeding.
- Send contents of uterine evacuation to the laboratory for analysis.

HYPEREMESIS GRAVIDARUM
Key signs and symptoms
- Continuous, severe nausea and vomiting
- Dehydration
- Oliguria

Key test results
- Arterial blood gas analysis reveals metabolic alkalosis.
- Hemoglobin level and hematocrit are elevated.
- Serum potassium level reveals hypokalemia.

Key treatment
- Restoration of fluid and electrolyte balance

Key interventions
- Monitor fundal height and the client's weight.
- Provide small, frequent meals.
- Maintain I.V. fluid replacement and total parenteral nutrition.

HYPERTENSIVE DISORDERS OF PREGNANCY
Key signs and symptoms
Gestational hypertension
- Onset of hypertension without associated proteinuria after 20 weeks' gestation; blood pressure returns to baseline by 12 weeks' postpartum

Preeclampsia
- Hypertension plus proteinuria
- Three categories of preeclampsia
  - Mild preeclampsia: Blood pressure 140/90 mm Hg; 300 mg of proteinuria in 24 hours
  - Severe preeclampsia: Blood pressure 160/110 mm Hg; 5 gm of proteinuria in 24 hours; less than 500 ml of urine in 24 hours
    - Vision disturbances
    - Right upper quadrant tenderness
    - Fetal growth restriction
  - Eclampsia
    - Presence of new-onset grand mal seizures in a client with preeclampsia

Chronic hypertension
- Medically diagnosed hypertension exists before pregnancy
- Gestational hypertension doesn't resolve within 12 weeks of delivery
- Superimposed preeclampsia
- Chronic hypertension plus new-onset proteinuria or other signs and symptoms of preeclampsia

Key test results
- Blood chemistry reveals increased blood urea nitrogen, creatinine, and uric acid levels and elevated liver function studies.

Key treatments
- Bed rest in a left lateral position
- Delivery: with mild preeclampsia, when the fetus is mature and safe induction is possible; with severe preeclampsia regardless of gestational age
- High-protein diet with moderate sodium intake
- Fluid and electrolyte replacement balanced with output

(continued)

Antepartum care refresher (continued)

HYPERTENSIVE DISORDERS OF PREGNANCY (CONTINUED)
- With severe preeclampsia: antihypertensives, such as hydralazine or labetalol
- Corticosteroid: betamethasone to accelerate fetal lung maturation
- Magnesium sulfate to reduce the amount of acetylcholine produced by motor nerves, thereby preventing seizures

Key interventions
For all clients
- Assess the client for edema and proteinuria.
- Maintain seizure precautions.
- Encourage bed rest in a left lateral recumbent position.
- Monitor blood pressure.

For clients with severe preeclampsia
- Assess maternal blood pressure every 1 to 4 hours or more frequently if unstable.
- Be prepared to obtain a blood sample for typing and cross-matching.
- Keep calcium gluconate (antidote to magnesium sulfate) nearby for administration at first sign of magnesium sulfate toxicity (elevated serum levels, decreased deep tendon reflexes, muscle flaccidity, central nervous system depression, and decreased respiratory rate and renal function).

MULTIFETAL PREGNANCY
Key signs and symptoms
- More than one set of fetal heart sounds
- Uterine size greater than expected for dates

Key test results
- Alpha fetoprotein levels are elevated.
- Ultrasonography is positive for multifetal pregnancy.

Key treatments
- Bed rest if early dilation occurs or at 24 to 28 weeks' gestation
- Biweekly NST to document fetal growth, beginning at 28 weeks' gestation
- Increased intake of calories, iron, folate, and vitamins
- Ultrasound examinations monthly to document fetal growth

Key interventions
- Monitor fetal heart sounds.
- Monitor maternal vital signs and weight.
- Monitor cardiovascular and pulmonary status.

PLACENTA PREVIA
Key signs and symptoms
- Painless, bright red vaginal bleeding, especially during the third trimester

Key test results
- Early ultrasound evaluation reveals the placenta implanted in the lower uterine segment.

Key treatments
- Treatment based on gestational age, when first episode occurs, and amount of bleeding
- If gestational age less than 34 weeks, hospitalizing the client and restricting her to bed rest to avoid preterm labor
- Treatment of choice: surgical intervention (by cesarean deliver) depending on placental placement and maternal and fetal stability

Key interventions
- Don't perform rectal or vaginal examinations unless equipment is available for vaginal and cesarean delivery.

- pulmonic systolic and apical systolic murmurs resulting from decreased blood viscosity and increased blood flow
- increased femoral venous pressure caused by impaired circulation from the lower extremities (resulting from the pressure of the enlarged uterus on the pelvic veins and inferior vena cava)
- decreased cerebrospinal fluid space from enlargement of the vessels surrounding the spinal cord's dura mater
- increased fibrinogen levels (up to 50% at term) from hormonal influences
- increased levels of blood coagulation factors VII, IX, and X, leading to a hypercoagulable state

- increase of about 33% in total red blood cell (RBC) volume, despite hemodilution and decreasing erythrocyte count
- hematocrit (HCT) decrease of about 7%
- increase of 12% to 15% in total hemoglobin (Hb) level; this is less than the overall plasma volume increase, thus reducing Hb concentration and leading to physiologic anemia of pregnancy
- leukocyte production equal to or slightly greater than blood volume increase (average leukocyte count is 10,000 to 11,000/µl; peaks at 25,000/µl during labor, possibly through an estrogen-related mechanism).

Cravings and more

GI system changes include:
- gum swelling from increased estrogen levels; gums may be spongy and bleed easily
- lateral and posterior displacement of the intestines
- superior and lateral displacement of the stomach
- delayed intestinal motility and gastric and gallbladder emptying time from smooth-muscle relaxation caused by high placental progesterone levels, causing heartburn
- nausea and vomiting (usually subside after the first trimester)
- hemorrhoids late in pregnancy from venous pressure
- constipation from increased progesterone levels, resulting in increased water absorption from the colon
- displacement of the appendix from McBurney point (making diagnosis of appendicitis difficult)
- bile saturation with cholesterol, sometimes leading to gallstone formation.

Hormonal changes

Endocrine system changes include:
- increased basal metabolic rate (up 25% at term) caused by demands of the fetus and uterus and by increased oxygen consumption
- increased iodine metabolism from slight hyperplasia of the thyroid caused by increased estrogen levels
- slight hyperparathyroidism from increased requirement for calcium and vitamin D
- elevated plasma parathyroid hormone levels, peaking between 15 and 35 weeks' gestation
- slightly enlarged pituitary gland
- increased production of prolactin by the pituitary gland late in pregnancy
- increased estrogen levels and hypertrophy of the adrenal cortex
- increased cortisol levels to regulate protein and carbohydrate metabolism
- possibly decreased maternal blood glucose levels
- decreased insulin production early in pregnancy
- increased production of estrogen, progesterone, and human chorionic somatomammotropin by the placenta and increased

levels of maternal cortisol, which reduce the mother's ability to use insulin, thus ensuring an adequate glucose supply for the fetus and placenta.

Altered breathing

Respiratory system changes include:
- increased vascularization of the respiratory tract caused by increased estrogen levels
- compression of the lungs caused by the enlarging uterus
- upward displacement of the diaphragm by the uterus
- increased tidal volume, causing slight hyperventilation
- increased chest circumference (by about 2⅜" [6 cm])
- altered breathing, with abdominal breathing replacing thoracic breathing as pregnancy progresses
- slight increase (2 breaths/minute) in respiratory rate
- lowered threshold for carbon dioxide due to increased levels of progesterone.

Everything increases

Metabolic system changes include:
- increased water retention caused by higher levels of steroidal sex hormones, decreased serum protein levels, and increased intracapillary pressure and permeability
- increased levels of serum lipids, lipoproteins, and cholesterol
- increased iron requirements caused by fetal demands
- increased carbohydrate needs
- increased protein retention from hyperplasia and hypertrophy of maternal tissues
- weight gain of 25 to 35 lb (11.3 to 16 kg). (See *What causes weight gain in pregnancy?*)

Is it getting hot in here?

Integumentary system changes include:
- hyperactive sweat and sebaceous glands
- changing pigmentation from the increase of melanocyte-stimulating hormone caused by increased estrogen and progesterone levels (darkened line from symphysis pubis to umbilicus known as linea nigra)
    - darkened nipples, areola, cervix, vagina, and vulva

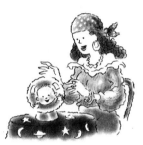

The future is clear. Pregnancy will affect nearly every body system.

What causes weight gain in pregnancy?

The following factors are responsible for the weight gain that occurs during pregnancy:
- fetus (7.5 lb [3.4 kg])
- placenta and membranes (1.5 lb [0.7 kg])
- amniotic fluid (2 lb [0.9 kg])
- uterus (2.5 lb [1.1 kg])
- breasts (3 lb [1.4 kg])
- blood volume (2 to 4 lb [0.9 to 1.8 kg])
- extravascular fluid and fat reserves (4 to 9 lb [1.8 to 4.1 kg])

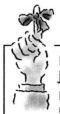

Attending to the client's increased nutritional needs can help prevent complications. Nutritional care is especially important for pregnant adolescents.

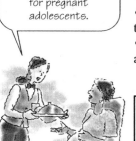

– pigmentary changes on nose, cheeks, and forehead known as facial chloasma
• striae gravidarum, commonly known as *stretch marks*, caused by weight gain and enlarged uterus.

Time to go (often)

Changes to the genitourinary system include:
• dilated ureters and renal pelvis caused by progesterone and pressure from the enlarging uterus, increasing the risk of urinary tract infection (UTI)
• increased glomerular filtration rate (GFR) and renal plasma flow (RPF) early in pregnancy; elevated GFR until delivery, but a near-normal RPF by term
• increased clearance of urea and creatinine from increased renal function
• decreased blood urea and nonprotein nitrogen values from increased renal function
• glycosuria from increased glomerular filtration without an increase in tubular reabsorptive capacity
• decreased bladder tone, causing urinary urgency and frequency
• increased sodium retention from hormonal influences
• increased dimensions of uterus
• hypertrophied uterine muscle cells (5 to 10 times normal size)
• increased vascularity, edema, hypertrophy, and hyperplasia of the cervical glands

• increased vaginal secretions with a pH of 3.5 to 6.0
• discontinued ovulation and maturation of new follicles
• thickening of vaginal mucosa, loosening of vaginal connective tissue, and hypertrophy of small-muscle cells. (See *Estimating delivery dates and gestational age.*)

Not just pickles and ice cream

Nutritional needs also change during pregnancy. For example:
• Calorie requirements during pregnancy exceed prepregnancy needs by 300 calories/day (from 2,100 to 2,400 calories/day).
• Protein requirements during pregnancy exceed prepregnancy needs by 30 g/day (from 46 to 76 g/day).
• Intake of all vitamins should increase, and a prenatal vitamin with iron is usually recommended.
• Folic acid intake is particularly important to help prevent fetal anomalies such as neural tube defects. Intake should be increased from 400 to 800 mg/day. Dietary sources of folic acid include green, leafy vegetables and whole-grain breads.
• Intake of all minerals, especially iron, should be increased. (See *Battling discomforts of pregnancy.*)
• Intake of fiber and fluid should be increased.

Estimating delivery dates and gestational age

• Nägele's rule determines the estimated date of delivery by subtracting 3 months from the first day of the last menses and adding 7 days; for example, October 5 − 3 months = July 5 + 7 days = July 12.
• Quickening is described as light fluttering fetal movement felt by the mother and is usually felt between 16 and 22 weeks' gestation.
• Fetal heart sounds can be detected with a Doppler ultrasound at 12 weeks' gestation and can be auscultated with a fetoscope at 16 to 20 weeks' gestation.

• Fetal crown-to-rump measurements, determined by ultrasound, can be used to assess the fetus's age until the head can be defined.
• Biparietal diameter is the widest transverse diameter of the fetal head. Measurements can be made by about 12 to 13 weeks' gestation.
• McDonald's rule uses fundal height in centimeters to determine the duration of pregnancy in weeks. To use this rule, place a tape measure at the symphysis pubis and measure up and over the fundus. Fundal height in centimeters $\times \ ^8/_7 =$ duration of pregnancy in weeks.

Battling discomforts of pregnancy

Education plays an important role in helping the client deal with discomforts.

FIRST-TRIMESTER DISCOMFORTS
Nausea and vomiting
Symptoms may occur at any time during pregnancy but are most prevalent during the first trimester. Teach the client to avoid greasy, highly seasoned foods; to eat small, frequent meals; and to eat dry toast or crackers before arising in the morning. Instruct the client to rise slowly from a lying or sitting position.

Nasal stuffiness, discharge, or obstruction
Advise the client to use a cool-mist vaporizer.

Breast enlargement and tenderness
Tell the client to wear a well-fitting support bra.

Urinary frequency and urgency
Instruct the client to decrease fluid intake in the evening to prevent nocturia, to avoid caffeine-containing fluids, and to respond to the urge to void immediately to prevent bladder distention and urinary stasis. Also teach the client how to perform Kegel exercises, and tell her to promptly report signs of urinary tract infections.

Fatigue
Tell the client to rest periodically throughout the day and to get at least 8 hours of sleep each night.

Increased leukorrhea
Advise the client to bathe daily and wear absorbent cotton underwear.

SECOND- AND THIRD-TRIMESTER DISCOMFORTS
Heartburn
Encourage the client to eat small, frequent meals; avoid fatty or fried foods; remain upright for at least 1 hour after eating; and use antacids that don't contain sodium bicarbonate.

Constipation
Encourage the client to exercise daily, increase fluid and dietary fiber intake, and maintain regular elimination patterns.

Hemorrhoids
Tell the client to avoid constipation, prolonged standing, and constrictive clothing, and advise her to use topical ointments, warm soaks, and anesthetic ointments to relieve symptoms.

Backache
Teach the client how to use proper body mechanics and maintain good posture. Also tell her to avoid wearing high heels.

Leg cramps
Instruct the client to increase calcium, frequently rest with legs elevated, wear warm clothing on the legs and, during a leg cramp, pull the toes up toward the leg while pressing down on the knee.

Shortness of breath
Encourage the client to maintain proper posture, especially when standing, and to sleep in semi-Fowler's position.

Ankle edema
Advise the client to wear loose-fitting garments, elevate the legs during rest periods, and ensure dorsiflexion of the feet if standing or sitting for prolonged periods.

Insomnia
Encourage the client to use relaxation techniques. Tell her to lie on her left side, using pillows to support her legs and abdomen.

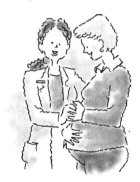

May I suggest you eat small, frequent meals and avoid fatty and fried foods.

Fetal development and structures

Structures unique to the fetus include fetal membranes, the umbilical cord, the placenta, and amniotic fluid.

His and her cells
Intrauterine development begins with **gametogenesis,** the production of specialized sex cells called *gametes.*

- The male gamete (spermatozoon) is produced in the seminiferous tubules of the testes during spermatogenesis.
- The female gamete (ovum) is produced in the graafian follicle of the ovary during oogenesis.
- As gametes mature, the number of chromosomes they contain is halved (through meiosis) from 46 to 23.

The moment of truth
Conception, or fertilization, occurs with the fusion of a spermatozoon and an

ovum (oocyte) in the ampulla of the fallopian tube.
- The fertilized egg is called a **zygote.**
- The diploid number of chromosomes (a pair of each chromosome; 44 autosomes and 2 sex chromosomes) is restored when the zygote is formed.
- A male zygote is formed if the ovum is fertilized by a spermatozoon carrying a Y chromosome.
- A female zygote is formed if the ovum is fertilized by a spermatozoon carrying an X chromosome.

A place to stay
Implantation occurs when the cellular wall of the blastocyst (trophoblast) implants itself in the endometrium of the anterior or posterior fundal region, about 7 to 9 days after fertilization.
- Primary villi appear within weeks after implantation.
- After implantation, the endometrium is called the *decidua.*

The beginning of the placenta
During **placental formation,** chorionic villi invade the decidua and become the fetal portion of the future placenta. By 4 weeks' gestation, a normal fetus begins to show noticeable signs of growth.

Fetal linings
Two fetal membranes are unique to the fetus:
- The **chorion** is the fetal membrane closest to the uterine wall; it gives rise to the placenta.
- The **amnion** is the thin, tough, inner fetal membrane that lines the amniotic sac.

Construction under way
Embryonic germ layers generate these fetal tissues:
- The **ectoderm** generates the epidermis, nervous system, pituitary gland, salivary glands, optic lens, lining of the lower portion of the anal canal, hair, and tooth enamel.

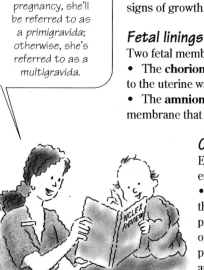

If this is the client's first pregnancy, she'll be referred to as a primigravida; otherwise, she's referred to as a multigravida.

- The **endoderm** generates the epithelial lining of the larynx, trachea, bladder, urethra, prostate gland, auditory canal, liver, pancreas, and alimentary canal.
- The **mesoderm** generates the connective and supporting tissues; the blood and vascular system; the musculature; teeth (except enamel); mesothelial lining of the pericardial, pleural, and peritoneal cavities; and kidneys and ureters.

The lifeline
The **umbilical cord** serves as the lifeline from the embryo to the placenta. At term, it measures from 20″ to 22″ (51 to 56 cm) in length and about ¾″ (2 cm) in diameter. The umbilical cord contains two arteries, one vein, and Wharton's jelly (which prevents kinking of the cord in utero). Blood flows through the cord at about 400 ml/minute.

Red on the outside, gray on the inside
The **placenta,** weighing about 1 to 1¼ lb (454 to 590 g) and measuring from 6″ to 10″ (15 to 25 cm) in diameter, contains 15 to 20 subdivisions called cotyledons and is 1″ to 1¼″ (2.5 to 3 cm) thick at term. Rough in texture, the placenta appears red on the maternal surface and shiny and gray on the fetal surface. The placenta:
- functions as a transport mechanism between the mother and the fetus
- has a life span and function that depends on oxygen consumption and maternal circulation; circulation to the fetus and placenta improves when the mother lies on her left side
- receives maternal oxygen by way of diffusion
- produces hormones, including human chorionic gonadotropin, human placental lactogen, gonadotropin-releasing hormone, thyrotropin-releasing factor, corticotropin, estrogen, and progesterone
- supplies the fetus with carbohydrates, water, fats, protein, minerals, and inorganic salts
- carries end products of fetal metabolism to the maternal circulation for excretion

• transfers passive immunity by way of maternal antibodies.

Fetal protection

The **amniotic fluid** prevents heat loss, preserves constant fetal body temperature, cushions the fetus, and facilitates fetal growth and development. Amniotic fluid is replaced every 3 hours.

At term, the uterus contains 800 to 1,200 ml of amniotic fluid, which is clear and yellowish and has a specific gravity of 1.007 to 1.025 and a pH of 7.0 to 7.25. Maternal serum provides amniotic fluid in early gestation, with increasing amounts derived from fetal urine late in gestation. Amniotic fluid contains:

• albumin
• bilirubin
• creatinine
• enzymes
• fat
• lanugo
• lecithin
• leukocytes
• sphingomyelin
• urea.

Blood movers

Fetal circulation structures include:
• one umbilical vein, which carries oxygenated blood to the fetus from the placenta
• two umbilical arteries, which carry deoxygenated blood from the fetus to the placenta
• the foramen ovale, which serves as the septal opening between the atria of the fetal heart
• the ductus arteriosus, which connects the pulmonary artery to the aorta, allowing blood to shunt around the fetal lungs
• the ductus venosus, which carries oxygenated blood from the umbilical vein to the inferior vena cava, bypassing the liver.

Keep abreast of diagnostic tests

Here's a brief review of tests performed as part of antepartum care.

The routine

These routine laboratory tests can confirm pregnancy and reveal maternal complications:
• **blood type, Rh, and abnormal antibodies** to identify the fetus at risk for erythroblastosis fetalis or hyperbilirubinemia
• **immunologic tests** such as rubella antibodies to detect the presence of rubella, rapid plasma reagin to detect untreated syphilis, hepatitis B surface antigen to detect hepatitis B, and human immunodeficiency virus (HIV) antibodies to detect HIV infection
• **urine tests** to detect UTI and to measure human chorionic gonadotropin (HCG) to confirm pregnancy
• **hematologic studies,** in which blood samples are used to analyze and measure RBCs, white blood cells (WBCs), erythrocyte sedimentation rate, platelets, Hb level, and HCT
• **coagulation studies,** in which a blood sample is used to analyze and measure prothrombin time (PT), partial thromboplastin time (PTT), and International Normalized Ratio (INR)
• **genital cultures,** such as a gonorrhea smear and chlamydia test, to detect sexually transmitted disease (STD)
• **triple screen** between 15 and 20 weeks' gestation to identify if the fetus is at increased risk for Down syndrome and neural tube defects
• **alpha fetoprotein,** which involves using a blood sample to measure alpha fetoprotein levels (high maternal serum levels may suggest fetal neural tube defects, such as spina bifida and anencephaly).

Nursing actions

Before the procedure
• Explain the procedure to the client.
After the procedure
• Check the venipuncture site for bleeding if blood was drawn.
• Label the specimen and send it to the laboratory.

Check your fluid?

Amniocentesis is usually performed after 14 weeks' gestation, when amniotic fluid is

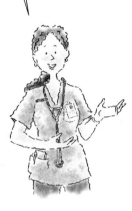

After amniocentesis, monitor the client for hemorrhage, infection, premature labor, and amnionitis.

sufficient and the uterus has moved into the abdominal cavity. This procedure involves transabdominal insertion of a spinal needle into the uterus to aspirate amniotic fluid. This procedure helps determine:
- gestational age by way of a lecithin-sphingomyelin ratio
- fetal lung maturity by analyzing lecithin-sphingomyelin ratio, two key components of surfactant
- creatinine levels.

Amniocentesis is used to diagnose genetic disorders, such as chromosomal aberrations, sex-linked disorders, inborn errors of metabolism, and neural tube defects. It may also be used to diagnose and evaluate isoimmune disorders, including Rh sensitization and ABO blood type incompatibility.

Nursing actions
Before the procedure
- Explain the procedure to the client.
- Make sure informed, written consent is obtained.

After the procedure
- Monitor the fetal heart rate (FHR) and uterine activity with an external fetal or fetal uterine monitor for several hours.
- Monitor for maternal hemorrhage, infection, premature labor, fetal hemorrhage, and amnionitis.
- Administer $Rh_O(D)$ immune globulin (RhoGAM) to Rh-negative mothers to prevent fetal isoimmunization.

Tissue sample
Chorionic villi sampling can be performed as early as 8 weeks' gestation. It involves removal and analysis of a small tissue specimen from the fetal portion of the placenta. This test helps determine the genetic makeup of the fetus, providing earlier diagnosis and allowing earlier and safer abortion if the fetus carries the risk of spontaneous abortion, infection, hematoma, fetal limb defects, and intrauterine death.

Nursing actions
Before the procedure
- Explain the procedure to the client.

You guessed it...the nonstress test doesn't bother me at all.

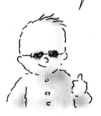

After the procedure
- Administer RhoGAM to Rh-negative mothers to prevent Rh sensitization.
- Monitor the FHR and uterine activity with an external fetal monitor for several hours.

Sound picture
Ultrasound, a painless procedure, uses ultrasonic waves reflected by tissues of different densities to visualize deep structures of the body. Reflected signals are then amplified and processed to produce a visual display, providing immediate results without harm to the fetus or mother. It may be performed vaginally, if necessary. Ultrasound can detect fetal death, malformation, or malpresentation; placental abnormalities; multiple gestation; and hydramnios or oligohydramnios. It's used to monitor fetal growth and estimate gestational age.

Nursing actions
Before the procedure
- Explain the procedure to the client.
- Instruct the client to drink a glass of water every 15 minutes, beginning 1½ hours before the procedure.
- Instruct the client not to void until immediately after the procedure.
- If the vaginal approach is necessary, instruct the client to void before the procedure and to avoid fluids.

After the procedure
- Offer a damp cloth to remove the conduction gel used to perform the study.

Stress-free
The **nonstress test** (NST) is used to detect fetal heart accelerations in response to fetal movement. This noninvasive test provides simple, inexpensive, immediate results without contraindications or complications. It may be indicated for a client at risk for uteroplacental insufficiency or for altered fetal movements.

The NST can be given between 32 and 34 weeks' gestation. A nonreactive test result indicates the possibility of fetal hypoxia, fetal sleep cycle, or the effects of drugs. The results may be inconclusive if the client is extremely obese.

Nursing actions
Before the procedure
- Explain the procedure to the client.
- Advise the client to eat a snack before testing.

After the procedure
- Allow the client to resume normal activities.

Contraction action
The **oxytocin challenge test** (OCT) evaluates fetal ability to withstand an oxytocin-induced contraction. This test, given after a nonreactive NST result, requires I.V. administration of oxytocin in increasing doses every 15 to 20 minutes until three high-quality uterine contractions are obtained within 10 minutes.

The OCT is performed on a client at risk for uteroplacental insufficiency or fetal compromise from diabetes, heart disease, hypertension, or renal disease or on a client with a history of stillbirth. The OCT isn't indicated for those with previous classic cesarean delivery or third-trimester bleeding or for those at high risk for preterm labor.

Nursing actions
Before the procedure
- Explain the procedure to the client.

During and after the procedure
- Monitor the FHR and uterine contractions with an external fetal monitor.

Breast test
The **nipple stimulation stress test** induces contractions by activating sensory receptors in the areola, triggering the release of oxytocin by the posterior pituitary gland. The receptors are activated by rolling the nipple manually or by applying a warm washcloth. This test has the same reactive pattern as the reactive NST result.

Nursing actions
Before the procedure
- Explain the procedure to the client.

During and after the procedure
- Monitor the FHR and uterine contractions with an external fetal monitor.

Good vibrations
The **vibroacoustic stimulation** test uses vibration and sound to induce fetal reactivity during an NST. Vibration is produced by an artificial larynx or a fetal acoustic stimulator (over the fetus's head for 1 to 5 seconds). This test is noninvasive, quick, and convenient.

Nursing actions
Before the procedure
- Explain the procedure to the client.

During and after the procedure
- Monitor the FHR with an external fetal monitor.

Six profiles in one
The **biophysical profile** assesses four to six parameters — fetal breathing movements, body movements, muscle tone, amniotic fluid volume, heart rate reactivity, and placental grade — using real-time ultrasound. This test is noninvasive and quick and can detect central nervous system (CNS) depression.

Nursing actions
Before the procedure
- Explain the procedure to the client.

During and after the procedure
- Monitor the FHR with an external fetal monitor.

How does the flow go?
Fetal blood flow studies use umbilical or uterine Doppler velocimetry to evaluate vascular resistance, especially in a client with hypertension, diabetes, isoimmunization, or lupus. These studies are useful when congenital anomalies or cardiac arrhythmias are suspected.

Nursing actions
Before and during the procedure
- Explain the procedure to the client.
- Before the procedure, obtain a baseline FHR.
- During the procedure, continue to monitor the mother and fetus for signs of problems, such as changes in vital signs or FHR or continuation of uterine contractions.

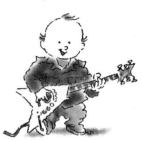

Vibroacoustic stimulation...I dig it!

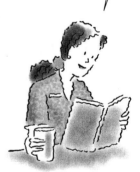

Put it together. Determination and knowledge. That's what you need to pass the exam.

Risky business

Percutaneous umbilical blood sampling (PUBS) is an invasive procedure that involves inserting a spinal needle into the umbilical cord to obtain fetal blood samples or to transfuse blood to the fetus in utero.

Usually performed during the second or third trimester, PUBS is indicated when the fetus is at risk for congenital and chromosomal abnormalities, congenital infection, or anemia. It carries a 1% to 2% risk of fetal loss.

Nursing actions

Before the procedure
- Explain the procedure to the client.
- Obtain a signed informed consent for the procedure.

During and after the procedure
- Monitor fetal and maternal status throughout the procedure.
- Administer RhoGAM to an Rh-negative mother after PUBS to prevent sensitization.

Every kick counts

Fetal movement count identifies the presence and frequency of fetal movement. Normally, fetal movement occurs about 280 times per day. Decreased movement may indicate fetal compromise.

Nursing actions

Before the procedure
- Explain the procedure to the client.
- Teach the client to record fetal movement for 30 minutes three times per day.
- Instruct the client to report fewer than 10 movements in 2 hours.

Polish up on client care

Potential antepartum complications and accompanying conditions include acquired immunodeficiency syndrome (AIDS), adolescent pregnancy, diabetes mellitus, ectopic pregnancy, heart disease, hydatidiform mole, hyperemesis gravidarum, hypertensive disorders of pregnancy, multifetal pregnancy, and placenta previa.

Acquired immunodeficiency syndrome

A female client may be first identified as positive for HIV antibodies during pregnancy or when the neonate's HIV status is identified. Because of the effects of pregnancy on immunosuppression, the progression from HIV infection to full-blown AIDS may be expedited during pregnancy.

CAUSES
- Exposure to HIV through blood transfusions, contaminated needles, or handling of blood
- Exposure to semen or vaginal secretions containing HIV

ASSESSMENT FINDINGS
- Diarrhea
- Fatigue
- HIV-associated dementia
- Kaposi's sarcoma
- Mild flulike symptoms
- Night sweats
- Opportunistic infections, such as toxoplasmosis, oral and vaginal candidiasis, herpes simplex, *Pneumocystis jiroveci* pneumonia, and *Candida* esophagitis
- Anorexia and weight loss

DIAGNOSTIC TEST RESULTS
- Blood chemistry shows increased transaminase, alkaline phosphatase, and gamma globulin level and decreased albumin level.
- CD4+ T-cell level is less than 200 cells/µl.
- Enzyme-linked immunosorbent assay shows positive HIV antibody titer.
- Hematology shows decreased WBC, RBC, and platelet counts.
- Western blot test is positive.

NURSING DIAGNOSES
- Fear
- Fatigue
- Ineffective protection
- Anxiety
- Ineffective coping

TREATMENT
- Care during pregnancy and delivery same as that for any other client with HIV
- Fetus monitored closely; serial ultrasounds performed to identify intrauterine growth restrictions; NST performed weekly after 32 weeks' gestation

Drug therapy
- If the client is newly diagnosed, zidovudine (Retrovir)or didanosine (Videx) is typically initiated at 14 to 34 weeks' gestation

INTERVENTIONS AND RATIONALES
- Assess for fever, chest tightness, and shortness of breath *to evaluate for possible recurrent acute pneumonia or pulmonary tuberculosis, which may indicate AIDS.*
- Administer total parenteral nutrition (TPN), if necessary, *to improve and support nutritional status.*
- Provide rest periods *to prevent fatigue.*
- Provide emotional support to the client and her family *to allay her fears.*
- Assess whether the client can care for her infant after delivery *to evaluate the need for additional support services.*

Teaching topics
- Explanation of the disorder and treatment plan
- Medication use and possible adverse effects
- Preventing the spread of infection
- Decreasing the risk of transmission to the fetus by avoiding unsafe sex practices or discontinuing I.V. drug use
- Counseling the client to help her decide whether to terminate the pregnancy

Adolescent pregnancy

A pregnant teenager is at risk for such complications as hypertensive disorders of pregnancy, cephalopelvic disproportion, anemia, and nutritional deficiencies. Teenagers also have a high incidence of STDs, posing a concern for both mother and neonate.

Infants born to teenagers are at risk for such complications as prematurity and low birth weight.

CONTRIBUTING FACTORS
- Peer pressure to be sexually active
- Desire to gain love, adulthood, and independence through pregnancy
- Fear of reporting sexual activity to parents
- High level of adolescent sexual activity
- Lack of appropriate role models
- Limited access to contraceptives
- Low level of education correlated with incorrect use of contraceptives
- Sporadic use of contraceptives
- Naiveté about ability to become pregnant

ASSESSMENT FINDINGS
- Amenorrhea
- Denial of pregnancy, which may deter the adolescent from seeking medical attention early in pregnancy

DIAGNOSTIC TEST RESULTS
- Pregnancy test is positive.
- Ultrasound confirms presence of fetus.

NURSING DIAGNOSES
- Deficient knowledge (pregnancy and care options)
- Imbalanced nutrition: Less than body requirements
- Interrupted family processes
- Fear

TREATMENT
- Diet with caloric intake sufficient to support the growing adolescent and her developing fetus
- Regular prenatal checkups

Drug therapy
- Antibiotics for STDs, if necessary
- Prenatal vitamins with iron

INTERVENTIONS AND RATIONALES
- Monitor the adolescent's weight gain *to assess for nutritional deficiencies.*
- Assess the adolescent's knowledge of her pregnancy *to determine the need for further teaching.*

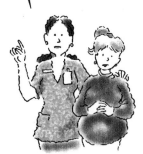

Be aware! Teenage mothers are at risk for insufficient or delayed medical care.

- Collect data about the adolescent's family and available support *to determine the need for referrals.*
- Provide nutritional support and encouragement *to promote the well-being of the mother and fetus.*
- Stress the importance of attending scheduled prenatal appointments *to promote the well-being of mother and fetus.*
- Advise the adolescent of her options, including terminating the pregnancy, continuing the pregnancy and giving up the infant for adoption, or continuing the pregnancy and keeping the infant, *to promote informed decision making.*
- Allow the adolescent to express her feelings about her pregnancy and herself *to promote mental and emotional well-being.*

Teaching topics
- Condition and any identified complications and the treatment plan
- Encouraging attendance at prenatal and birthing classes and infant care classes
- Recognizing the importance of prenatal care

Diabetes mellitus

In gestational diabetes mellitus, the client's pancreas, stressed by the normal adaptations to pregnancy, can't meet the increased demands for insulin.

A client may have preexisting diabetes or may develop gestational diabetes while she's pregnant. Gestational diabetes is associated with an increased risk of congenital anomalies, hydramnios, macrosomia, hypertensive disorders of pregnancy, spontaneous abortion, and fetal death. Additionally, the infant of a client with diabetes is at risk for developing sacral agenesis, a congenital anomaly characterized by incomplete formation of the vertebral column.

The client with gestational diabetes has an increased risk of developing diabetes mellitus at a later time.

RISK FACTORS
- Family history of diabetes
- Gestational diabetes in previous pregnancies

- Maternal age older than 25
- Obesity

ASSESSMENT FINDINGS
- Glycosuria
- Ketonuria
- Polydipsia
- Polyphagia
- Polyuria
- Fatigue
- Acetone breath
- Possible monilial infection (vaginal yeast infection)
- Possible UTI

DIAGNOSTIC TEST RESULTS
- One-hour glucose tolerance test reveals glucose level greater than 140 mg/dl.
- Three-hour glucose tolerance test reveals fasting serum glucose level of 105 mg/dl or greater.
- Three-hour glucose tolerance test reveals 1-hour serum glucose level of 190 mg/dl or greater.
- Three-hour glucose tolerance test reveals 2-hour serum glucose level of 165 mg/dl or greater.
- Three-hour glucose tolerance test reveals 3-hour serum glucose level of 145 mg/dl or greater.

NURSING DIAGNOSES
- Imbalanced nutrition: More than body requirements
- Risk for deficient fluid volume
- Ineffective coping
- Fear
- Anxiety

TREATMENT
- Monitoring of capillary blood sugar
- Exercise
- 1,800- to 2,200-calorie diet, divided into three meals and three snacks that should also include low fat and cholesterol and high fiber

Drug therapy
- Insulin or glyburide (DiaBeta) after the first trimester
- Other oral antidiabetic agents contraindicated because of adverse effects on the fetus

INTERVENTIONS AND RATIONALES
- Encourage adherence to dietary regulations *to maintain euglycemia.*
- Encourage the client to exercise moderately *to reduce blood glucose levels and decrease the need for insulin.*
- Prepare the client for antepartum fetal surveillance testing, including OCT, nipple stimulation stress testing, amniotic fluid index, biophysical profile, and NST, *to assess fetal well-being.*
- Encourage the client to verbalize her feelings *to allay her fears.*
- Provide emotional support *to reduce anxiety.*

Teaching topics
- Explanation of the disorder and treatment plan
- Medication use and possible adverse effects
- Performing capillary glucose monitoring
- Performing fetal "kick counts" to assess fetal well-being during the third trimester

Ectopic pregnancy

Ectopic pregnancy refers to implantation of the fertilized ovum outside the uterine cavity. Most commonly, ectopic pregnancy occurs in a fallopian tube; other sites include the cervix, ovary, and abdominal cavity. It's the second most frequent cause of vaginal bleeding early in pregnancy.

CAUSES
- Hormonal factors
- Malformed fallopian tubes
- Ovulation induction drugs
- Progestin-only hormonal contraceptives
- Tubal atony
- Tubal damage from pelvic inflammatory disease
- Tubal damage from previous pelvic or tubal surgery
- Tubal spasms
- Use of intrauterine devices

ASSESSMENT FINDINGS
- Hypotension
- Irregular vaginal bleeding; possible amenorrhea followed by bleeding
- Abdominal or pelvic pain; may be sharp or dull
- Nausea and vomiting
- Rapid, thready pulse
- Rupture of tubes, causing sudden and severe abdominal pain, syncope, and referred shoulder pain as the abdomen fills with blood
- Shock with profuse hemorrhage
- Uterine size smaller than expected for gestational age

DIAGNOSTIC TEST RESULTS
- HCG titers are abnormally low when compared to a normal pregnancy.
- Ultrasound is positive for ruptured tube and collective pelvic fluid.
- Vaginal examination reveals a palpable tender mass in Douglas' cul-de-sac.
- Serum progesterone levels are lower than in a normal pregnancy.

NURSING DIAGNOSES
- Deficient fluid volume
- Risk for infection
- Acute pain
- Fear

TREATMENT
- Laparotomy to ligate the bleeding vessels and remove or repair damaged fallopian tube
- Transfusion therapy: packed RBCs (if bleeding is uncontrolled)

Drug therapy
- If the tube hasn't ruptured, methotrexate (Trexall) followed by leucovorin to stop trophoblastic cells from growing (therapy continues until negative HCG levels are achieved)

INTERVENTIONS AND RATIONALES
- Monitor vital signs and intake and output *to assess for intense blood loss and shock.*
- Monitor for severe abdominal pain, orthostatic hypotension, tachycardia, and dizziness, *which may indicate rupturing ectopic pregnancy.*
- Administer I.V. fluid *to compensate for blood loss.*
- Administer blood products and monitor closely during infusion *to detect adverse reactions.*

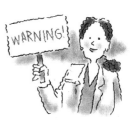

Severe abdominal pain, orthostatic hypotension, tachycardia, and dizziness may indicate a rupturing ectopic pregnancy.

WARNING!

- Administer RhoGAM *to combat isoimmunization in the client who's Rh-negative.*
- Provide routine postoperative care *to promote recovery.*
- Provide emotional support *for parents grieving over the loss of the pregnancy.*

Teaching topics

- Explanation of the disorder and treatment plan
- Medication use and possible adverse effects
- Importance of follow-up medical care

Heart disease

Heart disease occurs in about 1% of pregnant women. Pregnancy may reveal an underlying heart condition that previously produced no symptoms, or it may aggravate a known heart condition. A client with heart disease is at greatest risk when blood volume peaks between 28 and 32 weeks' gestation.

Successful delivery of a healthy baby depends on the type and extent of the disease. Decreased placental perfusion may lead to intrauterine growth retardation, fetal distress, and prematurity.

Pregnant clients with heart disease are graded as class I to IV.

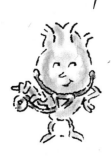

Pregnancy may reveal an underlying heart condition that previously produced no symptoms, or it may aggravate a known heart condition.

CAUSES

- Regurgitation, which permits blood to leak through an incompletely closed valve, thereby increasing the workload on heart chambers on either side of the affected valve
- Valvular stenosis (decreases blood flow through a valve, increasing workload on heart chambers located before the stenotic valve)

ASSESSMENT FINDINGS

- Tachycardia
- Dyspnea
- Fatigue
- Diastolic murmur at the heart's apex
- Crackles at the base of the lungs
- Cough
- Orthopnea
- Pitting edema
- Hemoptysis

DIAGNOSTIC TEST RESULTS

- Echocardiography, electrocardiogram (ECG), and chest X-ray may reveal cardiac abnormalities, impaired cardiac function, and cardiovascular decompensation.
- 12-lead ECG may reveal arrhythmias.

NURSING DIAGNOSES

- Activity intolerance
- Excess fluid volume
- Decreased cardiac output
- Ineffective breathing pattern

TREATMENT

- Low-sodium, low-fat diet with fluid restriction, if applicable
- Rest periods to prevent fatigue
- Oxygen therapy

Drug therapy

Class I and II
- Antibiotics: ampicillin (Omnipen-N), gentamicin to prevent bacterial endocarditis

Class III and IV
- Anticoagulant: heparin
- Antiarrhythmics: digoxin (Lanoxin), procainamide, beta-adrenergic blockers
- Antibiotics: ampicillin, gentamicin to prevent bacterial endocarditis
- Thiazide diuretics and furosemide (Lasix) to control heart failure if activity restriction and reduced sodium intake don't prevent it

INTERVENTIONS AND RATIONALES

- Monitor maternal and fetal vital signs *to assess for maternal and fetal well-being.*
- Assess cardiovascular and respiratory status *to assess for signs of maternal cardiac decompensation (tachycardia, tachypnea, moist crackles, exhaustion).*
- Administer anticoagulants, antiarrhythmics, antibiotics, and diuretics, as prescribed, *to achieve therapeutic regimens.*
- Encourage the client to monitor her intake *to avoid excessive weight gain.*
- Encourage the client to limit her physical activity according to her ability and symptoms *to ensure adequate rest.*
- Encourage the client to get 8 to 10 hours of sleep each night *to ensure adequate rest.*
- Monitor I.V. fluid intake and output *to maintain proper fluid levels.*

- Administer oxygen by nasal cannula or face mask during labor *to maintain fetal oxygenation.*
- Position the client on her left side with her head and shoulders elevated during labor *to prevent supine hypotension syndrome.*
- Continue to monitor the client during the postpartum period *to assess for signs of cardiac decompensation, even if distress is absent during pregnancy and labor.*

Teaching topics
- Explanation of the disorder and treatment plan
- Medication use and possible adverse effects
- Dietary modification
- Avoiding infection
- Recognizing signs and symptoms of heart failure
- Receiving adequate rest

Hydatidiform mole

Also known as *gestational trophoblastic disease,* hydatidiform mole is a developmental anomaly of the placenta that converts the chorionic villi into a mass of clear vesicles (hydatid vesicles). There are two types:
- *complete mole,* in which there's neither an embryo nor an amniotic sac
- *partial mole,* in which there's an embryo (usually with multiple abnormalities) and an amniotic sac.

CAUSES
- Possibly poor maternal nutrition or a defective ovum

ASSESSMENT FINDINGS
- Disproportionate enlargement of the uterus
- Excessive nausea and vomiting
- Intermittent or continuous bright red or brownish vaginal bleeding by 12 weeks' gestation
- Absence of fetal heart sounds
- Passage of clear, fluid-filled vesicles along with vaginal bleeding
- Symptoms of gestational hypertension before 20 weeks' gestation

DIAGNOSTIC TEST RESULTS
- HCG levels are extremely high for early pregnancy.
- Ultrasound fails to reveal a fetal skeleton.

NURSING DIAGNOSES
- Deficient fluid volume
- Complicated grieving
- Acute pain

TREATMENT
- Therapeutic abortion (suction and curettage) if a spontaneous abortion doesn't occur to prevent choriocarcinoma
- Pelvic examinations and chest X-rays at regular intervals
- Weekly monitoring of HCG levels until they remain normal for 3 consecutive weeks
- Periodic follow-up for 1 to 2 years because of increased risk of neoplasm

Drug therapy
- Methotrexate (Trexall) prophylactically (the drug of choice for choriocarcinoma)

INTERVENTIONS AND RATIONALES
- Monitor and record vital signs and intake and output *to assess for changes that may indicate complications.*
- Provide emotional support for the grieving couple *to demonstrate concern and understanding for the client and the family.*
- Monitor vaginal bleeding *to assess for hemorrhage.*
- Send contents of uterine evacuation to the laboratory for analysis *to assess for the presence of hydatid vesicles.*
- Advise the client to avoid pregnancy until HCG levels are normal (may take up to 2 years) *to avoid future complications.*

Teaching topics
- Explanation of the disorder and treatment plan
- Dealing with an uncertain obstetric and medical future
- Information on birth control

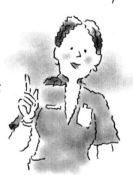

Hydatidiform mole is a chorionic tumor. The chorion is the fetal membrane closest to the uterine wall; it gives rise to the placenta.

Hyperemesis gravidarum

Hyperemesis gravidarum is persistent, uncontrolled vomiting that begins in the first weeks of pregnancy and may continue throughout pregnancy. Unlike "morning sickness," hyperemesis can have serious complications, including severe weight loss, dehydration, and electrolyte imbalance.

CAUSES
- Gonadotropin production
- Psychological factors
- Trophoblastic activity

ASSESSMENT FINDINGS
- Continuous, severe nausea and vomiting
- Dehydration
- Dry skin and mucous membranes
- Electrolyte imbalance
- Jaundice
- Metabolic alkalosis
- Nonelastic skin turgor
- Oliguria
- Significant weight loss

DIAGNOSTIC TEST RESULTS
- Arterial blood gas analysis reveals alkalosis.
- Hb level and HCT are elevated.
- Serum potassium level reveals hypokalemia.
- Urine ketone levels are elevated.
- Urine specific gravity is increased.

NURSING DIAGNOSES
- Imbalanced nutrition: Less than body requirements
- Deficient fluid volume
- Acute pain

TREATMENT
- TPN
- Restoration of fluid and electrolyte balance

Drug therapy
- Antiemetics, as necessary, for vomiting

INTERVENTIONS AND RATIONALES
- Monitor vital signs and fluid intake and output *to assess for fluid volume deficit.*
- Obtain blood samples and urine specimens *for laboratory tests, including Hb level, HCT, urinalysis, and electrolyte levels.*
- Monitor fundal height and the client's weight *to detect complications.*
- Provide small, frequent meals *to maintain adequate nutrition.*
- Maintain I.V. fluid replacement and TPN *to reduce fluid deficits and pH imbalances.*
- Provide emotional support *to help the client cope with her condition.*

Teaching topics
- Explanation of the disorder and treatment plan
- Recognizing triggers of nausea and vomiting
- Using salt on foods to replace sodium lost by vomiting

Hypertensive disorders of pregnancy

Hypertensive disorders of pregnancy include gestational hypertension, preeclampsia, chronichypertension, and superimposed hypertension. The client is at risk for cerebral hemorrhage, circulatory collapse, heart failure, hepatic rupture, and renal failure. If delivery occurs before term, the fetal prognosis is poor because of hypoxia, acidosis, and immaturity.

Maternal mortality from eclampsia is 10% to 15%, usually resulting from intracranial hemorrhage and heart failure.

RISK FACTORS
- Adolescence
- Antiphospholipid antibodies
- Diabetes mellitus
- Familial tendency
- Hydatidiform mole
- Hydramnios
- Hydrops fetalis
- Hypertension
- Malnutrition
- Maternal age older than 35
- Multifetal pregnancy
- Obesity
- Renal disease

A mother with gestational hypertension is at risk for cerebral hemorrhage, circulatory collapse, heart failure, hepatic rupture, and renal failure.

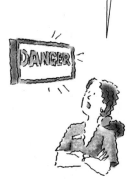

ASSESSMENT FINDINGS
Gestational hypertension
- Onset of hypertension without associated proteinuria after 20 weeks' gestation
- Blood pressure returning to baseline by 12 weeks' postpartum

Preeclampsia
- Hypertension plus proteinuria
- Three categories of preeclampsia
  - Mild preeclampsia
    - Blood pressure at least 140/90 mm Hg
    - 300 mg of proteinuria in 24 hours
    - Mild edema in upper extremities or face
  - Severe preeclampsia
    - Blood pressure 160/110 mm Hg
    - 5 gm of proteinuria in 24 hours
    - Less than 500 ml of urine in 24 hours
    - Vision disturbances
    - Pulmonary edema
    - Headaches, hyperreflexia, nausea
    - Right upper quadrant tenderness
    - Fetal growth restriction
    - Thrombocytopenia
  - Eclampsia
    - Presence of new-onset grand mal seizures in a client with preeclampsia

Chronic hypertension
- Medically diagnosed hypertension exists before pregnancy
- Gestational hypertension that doesn't resolve within 12 weeks of delivery
- Superimposed preeclampsia
- Chronic hypertension plus new-onset proteinuria or other signs and symptoms of preeclampsia

DIAGNOSTIC TEST RESULTS
- Blood chemistry reveals increased blood urea nitrogen, creatinine, and uric acid levels and elevated liver function studies.
- Hematology reveals thrombocytopenia (HELLP syndrome).

NURSING DIAGNOSES
- Activity intolerance
- Excess fluid volume
- Risk for injury
- Ineffective breathing pattern
- Decreased cardiac output

TREATMENT
- Bed rest in a left lateral position
- Delivery: with mild preeclampsia, when the fetus is mature and safe induction is possible; with severe preeclampsia, regardless of gestational age
- High-protein diet with moderate sodium intake
- Fluid and electrolyte replacement balanced with output

Drug therapy
- With severe preeclampsia: antihypertensives, such as hydralazine or labetalol
- Corticosteroid: betamethasone to accelerate fetal lung maturation
- Magnesium sulfate to reduce the amount of acetylcholine produced by motor nerves, thereby preventing seizures
- Diuretic: furosemide (Lasix) if pulmonary edema develops

INTERVENTIONS AND RATIONALES
For all clients
- Assess the client for edema and proteinuria, *which may indicate impending eclampsia.*
- Assess neurologic status *to detect early signs of deterioration, which might suggest impending eclampsia.*
- Monitor daily weight *to identify sodium and water retention.*
- Maintain a high-protein diet with moderate sodium restriction *as a measure against gestational hypertension.*
- Maintain seizure precautions *to ensure safety.*
- Encourage bed rest in a left lateral recumbent position *to improve uterine and renal perfusion.*
- Monitor blood pressure *to evaluate the effectiveness of treatment.*
- Monitor the FHR continuously during labor *to assess fetal well-being.*

For clients with severe preeclampsia
- Assess maternal blood pressure every 1 to 4 hours or more frequently if unstable *to assess for abnormalities.*
- If necessary, prepare for amniocentesis *to assess fetal maturity.*

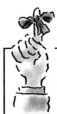

Memory jogger

Some women who develop preeclampsia also develop **HELLP** syndrome, so be alert if you notice the following signs:

Hemolysis

Elevated **L**iver enzyme levels

Low **P**latelet count.

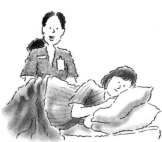

Encourage bed rest in a left lateral recumbent position to improve uterine and renal perfusion.

- Maintain I.V. fluids, as prescribed. *I.V. fluids are restricted based on urine output and total fluid intake per hour.*
- Obtain blood samples for complete blood count, platelet count, and liver function studies and to determine serum levels of blood urea nitrogen, creatinine, and fibrin degradation products *to detect signs of complications.*
- Be prepared to obtain a blood sample for typing and crossmatching *because of the risk of placenta previa.*
- Obtain urine specimens to determine urine protein levels and specific gravity, and perform 24-hour urine collection for protein and creatinine, as ordered, *to evaluate renal function.*
- Monitor urine output *to assess fluid status.*
- Keep calcium gluconate (antidote to magnesium sulfate) nearby *to administer at the first sign of magnesium sulfate toxicity* (elevated serum levels, decreased deep tendon reflexes, muscle flaccidity, CNS depression, and decreased respiratory rate and renal function).
- Promote relaxation *to reduce fatigue.*
- Encourage the client to verbalize her feelings *to allay anxiety.*
- Provide a quiet environment *to help prevent complications.*

Teaching topics
- Explanation of the disorder and treatment plan
- Importance of bed rest and adequate nutrition
- Recognizing signs and symptoms of severe preeclampsia and eclampsia

Multifetal pregnancy

A multifetal pregnancy, also known as *multiple gestation,* occurs when two or more embryos or fetuses exist simultaneously. Multifetal pregnancies are formed as follows:
- Single-ovum (monozygotic, identical) twins usually have one chorion, one placenta, two amnions, and two umbilical cords and are of the same sex.

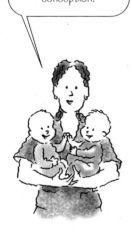

A multifetal pregnancy, also known as *multiple gestation,* may be either a single-ovum or double-ova conception.

- Double-ova (dizygotic, nonidentical) twins have two chorions, two placentas, two amnions, and two umbilical cords and may be of the same or different sex.
- Multifetal pregnancies of three or more fetuses may be single-ovum conceptions, multiple-ova conceptions, or a combination of both.

CAUSES
- In vitro fertilization
- Family history
- Gamete intrafallopian tube transfer
- Ovulation stimulation with such drugs as clomiphene (Clomid)

ASSESSMENT FINDINGS
- More than one set of fetal heart sounds
- Uterine size greater than expected for dates

DIAGNOSTIC TEST RESULTS
- Alpha fetoprotein levels are elevated.
- Ultrasonography is positive for multifetal pregnancy.

NURSING DIAGNOSES
- Anxiety
- Deficient knowledge (pregnancy)
- Risk for injury
- Fear

TREATMENT
- Activity, as tolerated, with increased rest periods
- Bed rest if early dilation occurs or at 24 to 28 weeks' gestation to improve uterine blood flow and, possibly, increase birth weight of the fetuses
- Biweekly NST to document fetal growth, beginning at 28 weeks' gestation
- Increased intake of calories, iron, folate, and vitamins
- Prenatal visits every 2 weeks, increasing to weekly between 24 and 28 weeks' gestation; cervical examinations performed at each visit to check for premature dilation
- Ultrasound examinations monthly to document fetal growth

INTERVENTIONS AND RATIONALES
- Monitor fetal heart sounds *to evaluate fetal well-being.*
- Monitor maternal vital signs and weight *to assess maternal well-being.*
- Monitor cardiovascular and pulmonary status *to assess for signs of gestational hypertension.*
- Ensure adequate nutrition and increased intake of folate, calories, vitamins, and iron *to ensure adequate weight gain.*
- Encourage frequent rest periods, especially during the third trimester, or to maintain bed rest, if indicated, *to prevent fatigue.*
- Provide emotional support and encouragement *to reduce anxiety.*
- Advise the client to return for ultrasound examination and NST as scheduled *to assess for fetal well-being.*

Teaching topics
- Pregnancy needs and expected course
- Notifying physician immediately if signs of premature labor occur
- Refraining from coitus during the third trimester

Placenta previa

In placenta previa, the placenta is implanted in the lower uterine segment (low implantation). The placenta can occlude the cervix partially or totally.

RISK FACTORS
- Maternal age older than 35
- Multiple pregnancies
- Placental villi torn from the uterine wall as the lower uterine segment contracts and dilates in the third trimester
- Uterine fibroid tumors
- Uterine scars from surgery
- Uterine sinuses exposed at the placental site and bleeding

ASSESSMENT FINDINGS
- Painless, bright red vaginal bleeding, especially during the third trimester (possibly increasing with each successive incident)

DIAGNOSTIC TEST RESULTS
- Early ultrasound evaluation reveals the placenta implanted in the lower uterine segment.

NURSING DIAGNOSES
- Fear
- Anxiety
- Deficient fluid volume
- Risk for injury

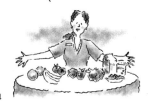

The nutritional needs of a client with a multifetal pregnancy exceed those of other pregnant women. Try some calories, iron, folate, and vitamins.

TREATMENT
- Treatment based on gestational age, when first episode occurs, and amount of bleeding
- If gestational age less than 34 weeks, hospitalizing the client and restricting her to bed rest to avoid preterm labor
- Administering supplemental iron if anemia is present
- Restricting maternal activities (for example, no lifting heavy objects, long-distance travel, or sexual intercourse)
- Transfusion of packed RBCs if Hb level and HCT are low
- Treatment of choice: surgical intervention (by cesarean delivery), depending on placental placement and maternal and fetal stability

INTERVENTIONS AND RATIONALES
- Monitor maternal vital signs, including uterine activity, *to assess maternal well-being.*
- Monitor for vaginal bleeding *to estimate blood loss.*
- Monitor for signs of infection; *clients with placenta previa are at increased risk for infection.*
- Monitor the FHR, using electronic fetal monitoring, *to assess for complications.*
- Don't perform rectal or vaginal examinations unless equipment is available for vaginal and cesarean delivery *to avoid stimulating uterine activity.*
- Obtain blood samples for HCT, Hb level, PT, INR, PTT, fibrinogen level, platelet count, and typing and crossmatching *to assess for complications.*
- Provide routine postoperative care if cesarean delivery is performed *to ensure the client's well-being.*
- Monitor for postpartum hemorrhage *because clients with placenta previa are more prone to hemorrhage.*

- Provide emotional support *to reduce anxiety.*
- Administer I.V. fluids, as ordered, *to reduce fluid loss.*
- Be prepared to administer betamethasone *to increase fetal lung maturity if preterm labor can't be halted.*

Teaching topics
- Explanation of the disorder and treatment plan
- Limiting activity
- Reporting increased bleeding immediately
- Understanding possible need for preterm delivery

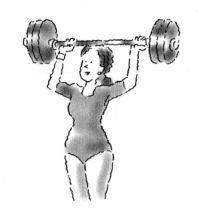

Pump up on practice questions

1. A 15-year-old client is 26 weeks pregnant. She has been admitted to the labor and delivery unit with a complaint of abdominal pain. Her parents want to speak with the nurse in reference to her condition. The nurse's best response to the parents is:
1. "I'll need a signed consent from your daughter to give you medical information."
2. "The physician can give you more information without consent."
3. "She'll be OK. It's just a stomachache."
4. "She's experiencing Braxton-Hicks contractions and is too young to understand the difference."

Answer: 1. A pregnant minor becomes emancipated to make decisions for herself and her baby. The client's right to confidentiality means that medical information of any kind can't be divulged without a signed consent from her. The physician can't give out information without consent.

➡ NCLEX keys
Client needs category: Safe and effective care environment
Client needs subcategory: Management of care
Cognitive level: Analysis

2. A client who's 32 weeks pregnant presents to the emergency department with bright red bleeding and no abdominal pain. Which action should the nurse take *first*?

1. Perform a pelvic examination.
2. Assess the client's blood pressure.
3. Assess the fetal heart rate (FHR).
4. Order a stat hemoglobin and hematocrit.

Answer: 3. The nurse should assess FHR for fetal distress or viability. A pelvic examination shouldn't be attempted because of the possibility of placenta previa, in which symptoms present as bright red bleeding without abdominal pain. The client's blood pressure should be addressed after fetal heart tones are attempted. Ordering a hemoglobin and hematocrit is a physician intervention, not a nursing intervention.

➡ NCLEX keys

Client needs category: Safe and effective care environment
Client needs subcategory: Management of care
Cognitive level: Analysis

3. Which finding is considered normal during the antepartum period of pregnancy?

1. Resting pulse rate fluctuations ranging from 15 to 20 beats/minute
2. Slight decrease in respiratory rate
3. Altered breathing pattern with thoracic breathing replacing abdominal breathing
4. Hematocrit (HCT) increase of about 7%

Answer: 1. Cardiovascular system changes associated with pregnancy lead to resting pulse rate fluctuation with increases ranging from 15 to 20 beats/minute at term. Other pregnancy-related changes include a slight increase (2 breaths/minute) in respiratory rate, altered breathing pattern with abdominal breathing replacing thoracic breathing as pregnancy progresses, and a decrease in HCT of about 7%.

➡ NCLEX keys

Client needs category: Health promotion and maintenance
Client needs subcategory: None
Cognitive level: Knowledge

4. A client comes to the clinic for her 12-week pregnancy checkup. The client asks the nurse when she should begin to feel her baby move. Which response should the nurse offer?

1. "You should have already felt it move."
2. "Typically women feel their baby move for the first time when they're 20 weeks pregnant."
3. "You'll probably feel your baby move after your 16th week of pregnancy."
4. "Each person experiences the baby's first movement at a different time throughout their pregnancy."

Answer: 3. Although each client does detect fetal movement at a different time, it's typically experienced just after the 16th week. If movement isn't detected around this time, problems with the pregnancy may exist.

➡ NCLEX keys

Client needs category: Health promotion and maintenance
Client needs subcategory: None
Cognitive level: Application

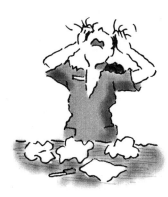

5. A client at a routine prenatal visit mentions to the nurse that she's nervous and afraid to go home. The nurse should respond by:

1. reassuring her that most new parents are nervous and that it's normal to feel this way.
2. contacting the admissions department to extend her stay.
3. asking her if she's unsafe at home.
4. excusing herself and reporting her remarks to the nurse in charge.

Answer: 3. The nurse has a legal responsibility to assess for and report abuse. False reassurance and extending her stay do not pinpoint the client's concern. The charge nurse may need to be notified after the nurse has defined the issue.

➡ *NCLEX keys*

Client needs category: Safe and effective care environment
Client needs subcategory: Management of care
Cognitive level: Application

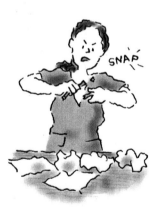

6. Which medication promotes fetal lung maturity in cases of preterm labor?
1. Terbutaline
2. Betamethasone
3. Co-trimoxazole (Bactrim)
4. Clarithromycin (Biaxin)

Answer: 2. Preterm labor raises concerns about the fetus's respiratory potential. Therefore, betamethasone is used to stimulate the development of surfactant in the lungs. Terbutaline is a beta-adrenergic agonist used to treat preterm labor. Co-trimoxazole is a sulfonamide commonly used to treat urinary tract infections, and clarithromycin is an antibiotic used to treat upper respiratory tract infections.

➡ *NCLEX keys*

Client needs category: Physiological integrity
Client needs subcategory: Pharmacological and parenteral therapies
Cognitive level: Application

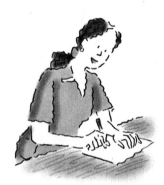

7. A multigravida client at 38 weeks' gestation has come to the emergency department complaining of chest pain. She tells the nurse that she has recently inhaled crack cocaine. The nurse's top priority is to assess the client for:
1. abruptio placentae.
2. placenta accreta.
3. malnutrition.
4. hypotension.

Answer: 1. The use of crack cocaine during pregnancy is associated with abruptio placentae, along with hypertension, stroke, tachycardia, hemorrhage, low birth weight, and preterm neonates. Crack cocaine isn't associated with placenta accreta (unusually deep attachment of the placenta to the uterine myometrium) or hypotension. Although malnutrition may exist, it isn't life-threatening at this point.

➥ NCLEX keys
Client needs category: Physiological integrity
Client needs subcategory: Reduction of risk potential
Cognitive level: Analysis

8. A multigravida client at 39 weeks' gestation is diagnosed with gestational hypertension and HELLP syndrome. The nurse's top priority is to assess the client's:
1. white blood count (WBC) count.
2. blood glucose levels.
3. serum iron levels.
4. platelet count.

Answer: 4. Women diagnosed with HELLP syndrome have hemolysis of red blood cells, elevated liver enzyme levels, and a low platelet count, so the nurse should assess the client's platelet count. This syndrome can lead to disseminated intravascular coagulation or hemorrhage. Monitoring WBC count, blood glucose levels, and serum iron levels isn't a priority for clients diagnosed with HELLP syndrome.

➥ NCLEX keys
Client needs category: Physiological integrity
Client needs subcategory: Reduction of risk potential
Cognitive level: Analysis

9. A hospitalized client who's 26 weeks pregnant has been diagnosed with gestational diabetes. She is overweight and doesn't understand the diet that has been suggested to her by the physician. The nurse asks the physician to order consults from which health care team member to demonstrate a gestational diabetic diet?
1. Social worker
2. Dietician
3. Psychologist
4. Lactation consultant

Answer: 2. A dietician can create a meal plan that will fit into the client's daily lifestyle and ensure specific calorie needs suggested by the physician. Dietary considerations will take into account the client's culture, food preferences, and activities of daily living. A social worker or psychologist would be consulted if psychological needs needed to be addressed. A lactation consultant could be consulted in the postpartum stage to address the client's and neonate's needs associated with breastfeeding.

➥ NCLEX keys
Client needs category: Safe and effective care environment
Client needs subcategory: Management of care
Cognitive level: Application

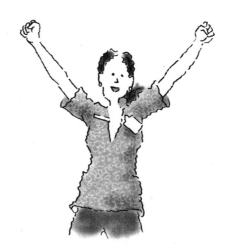

10. A nurse is performing a prenatal assessment on a client who's 32 weeks pregnant. She performs Leopold's maneuvers and

determines that the fetus is in the cephalic position. Identify where the nurse should place the Doppler to auscultate fetal heart tones.

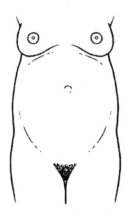

Answer: When the fetus is in the cephalic position (head down), fetal heart tones are best auscultated midway between the symphysis pubis and the umbilicus. When the fetus is in the breech position, fetal heart tones are best heard at or above the level of the umbilicus.

➡ *NCLEX keys*

Client needs category: Health promotion and maintenance
Client needs subcategory: None
Cognitive level: Analysis

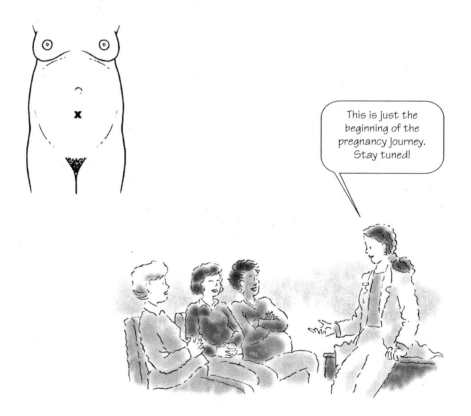

This is just the beginning of the pregnancy journey. Stay tuned!

4 Intrapartum care

In this chapter, you'll review:

✍ components and stages of labor

✍ how to perform maternal and fetal evaluations

✍ common complications of labor and delivery, such as preterm labor and prolapsed umbilical cord

✍ client care for such situations as preterm labor and cesarean birth.

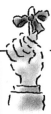

Memory jogger

To remember the three key components of labor, think of the 3 Ps:

Passage

Passenger

Power.

Brush up on key concepts

Intrapartum care refers to care of the client during labor. In this section, you'll find a brief review of the signs and symptoms that indicate the onset of labor, the client's physiologic and psychosocial responses to labor, basic obstetric procedures, and methods of monitoring the client and fetus.

At any time, you can review the major points of this chapter by consulting the *Cheat sheet* on pages 50 to 53.

Components of labor

The three major components of labor are the passage, the passenger, and the power. These components must work together for labor to progress normally.

Long and winding road
Passage refers to the maternal pelvis and soft tissues, the passageway through which the fetus exits the body. This area is affected by the shape of the inlet, the structure of the pelvis, and pelvic diameters.

Coach or first class?
Passenger refers to the fetus and its ability to move through the passage. This ability is affected by such fetal features as:
• the skull
• the lie (relationship of the long axis [spine] of the fetus to the long axis of the mother)
• presentation (portion of the fetus that enters the pelvic passageway first)
• position (relationship of the presenting part of the fetus to the front, back, and sides of the maternal pelvis).

Attitude refers to the relationship of the fetal parts (such as the chest, chin, or arms) to one another during the passage through the birth canal. The fetal head may be in a flexed (chin-to-chest) or extended (head-to-back) position. Pressure exerted by the maternal pelvis and birth canal during labor and delivery causes the sutures of the skull to allow the cranial bones to shift, resulting in molding of the fetal head.

What kind of engine?
Power refers to uterine contractions, which cause complete cervical effacement (thinning) and dilation (expansion).

Along for the ride
Other factors that affect labor are:
• accomplishment of the tasks of pregnancy
• coping mechanisms
• mother's ability to bear down (voluntary use of abdominal muscles to push during the second stage of labor)
• past experiences
• placental positioning
• preparation for childbirth
• psychological readiness
• support systems.

Let's get this show on the road
Preliminary signs that indicate the onset of labor may occur anywhere from 24 hours to 3 weeks before onset of true labor. They include:
• lightening, or fetal descent into the pelvis, which usually occurs 2 to 3 weeks before term in a primiparous client and later or during labor in a multiparous client
• Braxton Hicks contractions, which can occur irregularly and intermittently throughout pregnancy and may become uncomfortable and produce false labor

(Text continues on page 53.)

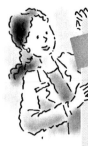

Cheat sheet

Intrapartum care refresher

ABRUPTIO PLACENTAE

Key signs and symptoms
- Acute abdominal pain and rigid abdomen
- Hemorrhage with dark red vaginal bleeding

Key test results
- Ultrasonography locates the placenta and may reveal a clot or hematoma.

Key treatments
- Transfusion: packed red blood cells (RBCs), platelets, and fresh frozen plasma, if necessary
- Cesarean birth

Key interventions
- Avoid pelvic or vaginal examinations and enemas.
- Administer blood products and monitor vital signs.
- Position the client in a left lateral recumbent position.

AMNIOTIC FLUID EMBOLISM

Key signs and symptoms
- Cyanosis and chest pain
- Tachypnea and sudden dyspnea

Key test results
- Electronic fetal monitor reveals fetal distress (during the intrapartum period).
- Arterial blood gas results reveal hypoxemia.

Key treatments
- Oxygen therapy: endotracheal intubation and mechanical ventilation if respiratory arrest occurs
- Cardiopulmonary resuscitation (CPR) if client is apneic and pulseless
- Emergency delivery by cesarean birth

Key interventions
- Assess respiratory and cardiovascular status.
- Assess fetal heart rate (FHR).
- Perform CPR, if necessary.
- Assist with immediate delivery of the neonate.

DISSEMINATED INTRAVASCULAR COAGULATION

Key signs and symptoms
- Abnormal bleeding (petechiae, hematomas, ecchymosis, cutaneous oozing)
- Oliguria

Key test results
- Coagulation studies reveal decreased fibrinogen level, positive D-dimer test specific for disseminated intravascular coagulation, prolonged prothrombin time (PT), and prolonged partial thromboplastin time (PTT).
- Hematology studies reveal decreased platelet count.

Key treatments
- Transfusion therapy: packed RBCs, fresh frozen plasma, platelets, and cryoprecipitate
- Treatment of the underlying condition
- Immediate delivery of the fetus by cesarean birth

Key interventions
- Monitor cardiovascular, respiratory, neurologic, GI, and renal status.
- Monitor vital signs frequently.
- Monitor intake and output.
- Administer blood products and monitor client closely for signs and symptoms of a transfusion reaction.
- Monitor the results of serial blood studies.

DYSTOCIA

Key signs and symptoms
- Arrested descent
- Hypotonic contractions

Key test results
- Ultrasonography shows fetal position or malformation or fetal weight greater than 4,500 g.

Key treatments
- Delivery of the fetus by cesarean birth if labor fails to progress and the mother or fetus shows signs of compromise
- Uterotonic: oxytocin (Pitocin) if contractions are ineffective

> I've got the power! Power, the passenger, and the passage make up the three major components of labor.

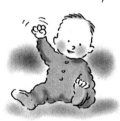

Intrapartum care refresher (continued)

DYSTOCIA (CONTINUED)
Key interventions
- Monitor maternal vital signs and FHR.
- Assist the patient to a left side-lying position.
- Monitor the effectiveness of oxytocin therapy, and watch for complications.

EMERGENCY BIRTH
Key signs and symptoms
For prolapsed umbilical cord
- Cord visible at the vaginal opening
- Variable decelerations or bradycardia noted on the fetal monitor strip

For uterine rupture
- Abdominal pain and tenderness, especially at the peak of a contraction, or the feeling that "something ripped"
- Excessive external bleeding
- Late decelerations, reduced FHR variability, tachycardia and bradycardia, and cessation of FHR
- Palpation of the fetus outside the uterus

For amniotic fluid embolism
- Chest pain
- Coughing with pink, frothy sputum
- Increasing restlessness and anxiety
- Sudden dyspnea
- Tachypnea

Key test results
For prolapsed umbilical cord
- Ultrasonography confirms that the cord is prolapsed.

For uterine rupture
- Ultrasonography may reveal the absence of the amniotic cavity within the uterus.

For amniotic fluid embolism
- Arterial blood gas analysis reveals hypoxemia.

Key treatments
- Administration of oxygen by nasal cannula or mask (endotracheal intubation and mechanical ventilation may be necessary in the case of amniotic fluid embolism)
- Emergency cesarean delivery

Key interventions
- Monitor maternal vital signs, pulse oximetry, and intake and output as well as FHR.
- Administer maternal oxygen by cannula or mask at 8 to 10 L/minute.
- Maintain I.V. fluid replacement.
- Place the client in a left lateral recumbent position.

- Obtain blood samples to determine hematocrit (HCT), hemoglobin (Hb) level, PT and PTT, fibrinogen level, and platelet count and to type and crossmatch blood.
- Monitor administration of blood products as necessary.
- Prepare the client and her family for the possibility of cesarean delivery.

FETAL DISTRESS
Key signs and symptoms
- Electronic fetal monitor showing bradycardia or FHR greater than 180 beats/minute
- Loss of fetal movement

Key test results
- Fetal scalp blood sampling reveals acidosis.

Key treatments
- Supplemental oxygen by face mask, typically at 6 to 8 L/minute
- I.V. fluid administration
- Emergency fetal delivery by vacuum aspiration, forceps, or cesarean birth

Key interventions
- Monitor FHR, fetal activity, and fetal heart variability.
- Assist the client to a left side-lying position.

INVERTED UTERUS
Key signs and symptoms
- Large, sudden gush of blood from the vagina
- Severe uterine pain

Key test results
- Hematology tests reveal decreased levels of Hb and HCT.

Key treatments
- Fluid resuscitation with I.V. fluids and blood products
- Supplemental oxygen administration
- Immediate manual replacement of the uterus
- Possible emergency hysterectomy
- Tocolytic agent: terbutaline

Key interventions
- Administer supplemental oxygen.
- Monitor vital signs frequently.
- Monitor intake and output.

LACERATION
Key signs and symptoms
- Increased vaginal bleeding after delivery of placenta

Key test results
- Hematology studies may reveal decreased levels of Hb and HCT.

(continued)

Intrapartum care refresher *(continued)*

LACERATION *(CONTINUED)*
Key treatments
- Laceration repair
- Analgesics: ibuprofen (Motrin), acetaminophen and oxycodone (Percocet), acetaminophen (Tylenol)

Key interventions
- Monitor vital signs, including temperature.
- Monitor laceration site for signs of infection and bleeding.
- Insert indwelling urinary catheter, if indicated.

PRECIPITATE LABOR
Key signs and symptoms
- Cervical dilation greater than 5 cm/hour in a nulliparous woman; more than 10 cm/hour in a multiparous woman

Key test results
- There are no diagnostic test findings specific to this complication.

Key treatments
- Controlled delivery to prevent maternal and fetal injury

Key interventions
- Monitor FHR and variability.

PREMATURE RUPTURE OF MEMBRANES
Key signs and symptoms
- Blood-tinged amniotic fluid gushing or leaking from the vagina
- Uterine tenderness

Key test results
- Vaginal probe ultrasonography allows detection of amniotic sac tear or rupture.

Key treatments
- Hospitalization to monitor for maternal fever and leukocytosis and fetal tachycardia if pregnancy is between 28 and 34 weeks. If infection is confirmed, labor must be induced.
- Oxytocic agent: oxytocin (Pitocin) for labor induction if term pregnancy and labor doesn't result within 24 hours after membrane rupture

Key interventions
- Assess for signs of infection or fetal distress.
- Administer antibiotics as prescribed.
- Encourage the client to express her feelings and concerns.

PRETERM LABOR
Key signs and symptoms
- Feeling of pelvic pressure or abdominal tightening
- Increased vaginal discharge

- Intestinal cramping
- Uterine contractions that result in cervical dilation and effacement

Key test results
- Electronic fetal monitoring confirms uterine contractions.
- Vaginal examination confirms cervical effacement and dilation.

Key treatments
- Betamethasone administered I.M. at regular intervals over 48 hours to increase fetal lung maturity in a fetus expected to be delivered preterm
- Tocolytic agents, such as terbutaline and ritodrine (Yutopar), to inhibit uterine contractions
- Magnesium sulfate to maintain uterine relaxation

Key interventions
- Monitor maternal vital signs, contractions, and FHR every 15 minutes during tocolytic therapy (otherwise, provide continuous fetal monitoring).
- Monitor for maternal adverse reactions to terbutaline or ritodrine.
- Monitor for magnesium sulfate toxicity, and make sure calcium gluconate is available.
- Assess the neonate for possible adverse affects of indomethacin (Indocin), such as premature closure of the ductus arteriosus.

PROLAPSED UMBILICAL CORD
Key signs and symptoms
- Cord visible at the vaginal opening
- Variable decelerations or bradycardia noted on the fetal monitor strip

Key test results
- Ultrasonography may reveal the cord as the presenting part.

Key treatments
- Immediate delivery of the fetus

Key interventions
- Place the client in Trendelenburg's position (position the woman's hips higher than her head in a knee-to-chest position).
- Monitor FHR and variability.

UTERINE RUPTURE
Key signs and symptoms
- Abdominal pain and tenderness, especially at the peak of a contraction, or the feeling that "something ripped"
- Late decelerations, reduced FHR variability, tachycardia and bradycardia, and cessation of FHR

Intrapartum care refresher *(continued)*

UTERINE RUPTURE *(CONTINUED)*

Key test results
• Hematology tests reveal decreased levels of Hb and HCT.

Key treatments
• Fluid resuscitation: I.V. fluids and blood products via rapid infusion

• Surgery to remove the fetus and repair the tear, or hysterectomy, if necessary
• Oxytocic agent: oxytocin (Pitocin) to help contract the uterus

Key interventions
• Monitor vital signs frequently.
• Prepare the client for immediate surgery.

• cervical changes, including softening, effacement, and slight dilation several days before the initiation of labor
• a sudden burst of energy before the onset of labor, commonly demonstrated by housecleaning activities and called the *nesting instinct* (See *True or false?*)
• bloody show as the mucus plug is expelled from the cervix
• increase in clear vaginal secretions
• rupture of membranes, occurring before the onset of labor in about 12% of clients and within 24 hours for about 80% of clients.

Evaluating the mother during true labor

Here's a review of methods and techniques used to monitor the progress of true labor and the mother's condition.

Starting to open
Observe **dilation.** The cervical os should increase from 0 to 10 cm.

The thick and thin of it
Observe **effacement,** cervical thinning and shortening, which is measured from 0% (thick) to 100% (paper thin).

What's the situation?
Using abdominal palpation (Leopold's maneuvers), determine **fetal position and presentation.** The process consists of four maneuvers.

Palpate the fundus to identify the occupying fetal part: the fetus's head is firm and rounded and moves freely; the breech is softer and less regular and moves with the trunk.

Palpate the abdomen to locate the fetus's back: the back should feel firm, smooth, and convex, whereas the front is soft, irregular, and concave.

Determine the level of descent of the head by grasping the lower portion of the abdomen above the symphysis pubis to identify the fetal part presenting over the inlet; an unengaged head can be rocked from side to side.

True or false?

Use the chart below to help distinguish between true and false labor.

True labor	False labor
Regular contractions	Irregular, brief contractions
Back discomfort that spreads to the abdomen	Discomfort that's localized in the abdomen
Progressive cervical effacement and dilation	No cervical change
Gradually shortened intervals between contractions	No change or irregular change in intervals between contractions
Increased intensity of contractions with ambulation	Contractions that may be relieved with ambulation
Contractions that increase in duration and intensity	Usually no change in duration and intensity of contractions
Usually bloody show	Usually no bloody show

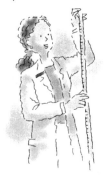

> Uterine contractions are measured by duration, frequency, and intensity.

Determine head flexion by moving fingers down both sides of the uterus to assess the descent of the presenting part into the pelvis; greater resistance is met as the fingers move downward on the cephalic prominence (brow) side.

What's the relationship?

Check the **station,** the relationship of the presenting part to the pelvic ischial spines:
- The presenting part is even with the ischial spines at 0 station.
- The presenting part is above the ischial spines at −3, −2, or −1.
- The presenting part is below the ischial spines at +1, +2, or +3.

Thirsty?

Monitor the client for signs of **dehydration,** such as poor skin turgor, decreased urine output, and dry mucous membranes.

I need a little rest

Use an external pressure transducer to monitor the client for **tetanic contractions,** sustained prolonged contractions with little rest in between that reduce oxygen supply to the fetus.

Measuring contractions

Phases of **uterine contractions** include increment (buildup and longest phase), acme (peak of the contraction), and decrement (letting-down phase). Contractions are measured by duration, frequency, and intensity. Here's how to measure each:
- **Duration** is measured from the beginning of the increment of the contraction to the end of the decrement of the contraction and averages 30 seconds early in labor and 60 seconds later in labor.
- **Frequency** is measured from the beginning of one contraction to the beginning of the next and averages 5 to 30 minutes apart early in labor and 2 to 3 minutes apart later in labor.
- **Intensity** is assessed during the acme phase and can be measured with an intrauterine catheter or by palpation; normal resting pressure when using an intrauterine catheter is 5 to 15 mm Hg; pressure increases to 30 to 50 mm Hg during the acme. When assessing intensity by palpation, the contraction is considered mild, moderate, or strong.

All around adaptations

Labor also prompts a series of responses throughout the mother's body, including changes in the cardiovascular, respiratory, and GI systems. (See *Maternal responses to labor.*)

Maternal responses to labor

During labor, the mother undergoes physiologic changes.

CARDIOVASCULAR SYSTEM
- Increased intrathoracic pressure during pushing in the second stage
- Increased peripheral resistance during contractions, which elevates blood pressure and decreases pulse rate
- Increased cardiac output

FLUID AND ELECTROLYTE BALANCE
- Increased water loss from diaphoresis and hyperventilation

- Increased evaporative water volume from increased respiratory rate

RESPIRATORY SYSTEM
- Increased oxygen consumption
- Increased respiratory rate

HEMATOPOIETIC SYSTEM
- Increased plasma fibrinogen level and leukocyte count
- Decreased blood coagulation time and blood glucose levels

GI SYSTEM
- Decreased gastric motility and absorption

- Prolonged gastric emptying time

RENAL SYSTEM
- Forward and upward displacement of the bladder base at engagement
- Possibly proteinuria from muscle breakdown
- Possibly impaired blood and lymph drainage from the bladder base, resulting from edema caused by the presenting fetal part
- Decreased bladder sensation if epidural anesthetic has been administered

Evaluating the fetus during true labor

Evaluation of uterine contractions and fetal heart rate (FHR) during true labor involves external and internal monitoring.

Heart check
FHR can be monitored either intermittently with a handheld device or continuously with an electronic fetal monitor.

Pressure check
Contraction frequency and intensity is monitored externally with a **tocotransducer.** This pressure-sensitive device records uterine motion during contractions. Contractions may also be monitored by palpation.

From the inside out
Internal electronic fetal monitoring can evaluate fetal status during labor more accurately than external methods. A spiral electrode attached to the presenting fetal part provides the baseline FHR and allows evaluation of FHR variability.

Intense info
To determine the true intensity of contractions, a **pressure-sensitive catheter** is inserted into the uterine cavity alongside the fetus.

Stages of labor

The labor process is divided into four stages, ranging from the onset of true labor through delivery of the fetus and placenta to the first hour after delivery.

FIRST STAGE
The first stage is measured from the onset of true labor to complete dilation of the cervix. This period lasts from 6 to 18 hours in a primiparous client and from 2 to 10 hours in a multiparous client. There are three phases of stage one.

This is getting exciting
During the **latent phase,** the cervix is dilated 0 to 3 cm, contractions are irregular, and the client may experience anticipation, excitement, or apprehension. Cervical effacement is almost complete.

This is getting serious
During the **active phase,** the cervix is dilated 4 to 7 cm. Cervical effacement is complete. Contractions are about 5 to 8 minutes apart and last 45 to 60 seconds with moderate to strong intensity. During this phase, the client becomes serious and concerned about the progress of labor; she may ask for pain medication or use breathing techniques. If membranes haven't ruptured spontaneously, amniotomy may be performed.

Whole lotta shakin' going on
During the **transitional phase,** the cervix is dilated 8 to 10 cm. Contractions are about 1 to 2 minutes apart and last 60 to 90 seconds with strong intensity. During this phase, the client may lose control, thrash in bed, groan, or cry out.

SECOND STAGE
The second stage of labor extends from complete dilation to delivery. This stage lasts an average of 40 minutes (20 contractions) for the primiparous client and 20 minutes (10 contractions) for the multiparous client. It may last longer if the client has had epidural anesthesia.

The client may become exhausted and dehydrated as she moves from coping with contractions to actively pushing. During this stage, the fetus is moved along the birth canal by the mechanisms of labor described here.

A brief engagement
The fetus's head is considered to be **engaged** when the biparietal diameter passes the pelvic inlet.

Going down
The movement of the presenting part through the pelvis is called **descent.**

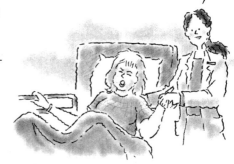

Remember that the client shouldn't try to push until the cervix is completely dilated.

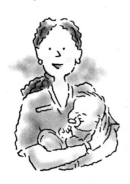

Helping to promote maternal-neonatal bonding is a key nursing responsibility in the first hour after delivery.

Nursing care during labor and delivery

Nursing actions include interventions that correspond to all stages of labor as well as those that apply only to certain stages.

CARE DURING ALL STAGES OF LABOR
• Monitor and record vital signs, I.V. fluid intake, and urine output.
• Provide emotional support to the client and her coach.
• Assess the need for pain medication, and evaluate the effectiveness of pain-relief measures.
• Maintain sterile technique and standard precautions.
• Maintain the client's comfort by offering mouth care, ice chips, and a change of bed linen.
• Explain the purpose of all nursing actions and medical equipment.

CARE DURING FIRST AND SECOND STAGES
• Monitor the frequency, duration, and intensity of contractions.

• Monitor fetal heart rate during and between contractions, and report changes.
• Observe for rupture of membranes, noting the time, color, odor, amount, and consistency of amniotic fluid.
• Watch for signs of hypotensive supine syndrome; if blood pressure falls, position the client on the left side and report changes immediately.
• During the second stage, observe the perineum for show and bulging.

CARE DURING FIRST, SECOND, AND THIRD STAGES
• Assist with breathing techniques.
• Encourage rest between contractions.

CARE DURING THE FOURTH STAGE
• Assess lochia and the location and consistency of the fundus.
• Encourage bonding.
• Initiate breast-feeding.

Flex that chin
During **flexion,** the head flexes so that the chin moves closer to the chest.

Head rotation I
Internal rotation is the rotation of the head in order to pass through the ischial spines.

Stretch as you go by
Extension is when the head extends as it passes under the symphysis pubis.

Head rotation II
External rotation involves the external rotation of the head as the shoulders rotate to the anteroposterior position in the pelvis.

THIRD STAGE
The third stage of labor extends from delivery of the neonate to expulsion of the placenta and lasts from 5 to 30 minutes.

Pain, then placenta
During this period, the client typically focuses on the neonate's condition. The client may experience discomfort from uterine contractions before expelling the placenta.

FOURTH STAGE
The fourth stage of labor is the 1 to 4 hours after delivery, when the primary activity is the promotion of maternal-neonatal bonding.

For a review of nursing actions during the delivery process, see *Nursing care during labor and delivery.*

Pain relief during labor and delivery

Pain relief is an important element of client care during labor and delivery. Pain relief during labor includes nonpharmacologic methods, analgesics, and general or regional anesthetics.

Just relax
Relaxation techniques may be effective.

Just rub it
Effleurage, a light abdominal stroking with the fingertips in a circular motion, is effective for mild to moderate discomfort.

Hey, look over here
Distraction can divert attention from mild discomfort early in labor. Focal point imaging and music are sometimes effective diversions.

Breathing, breathing, breathing
Three patterns of controlled chest breathing, called **Lamaze breathing,** are used primarily during the active and transitional phases of labor.

Ancient pain relief
The stimulation of key trigger points with needles (**acupuncture**) or finger pressure (**acupressure**) can reduce pain and enhance energy flow.

Pain relief but not without risk
Opioids, such as nalbuphine, can be used to relieve pain. If an opioid is given within 2 hours of delivery, it can cause neonatal respiratory depression, hypotonia, and lethargy.

Less pain but still awake
Lumbar epidural anesthesia requires an injection of medication into the epidural space in the lumbar region, leaving the client awake and cooperative. An epidural provides analgesia for the first and second stages of labor and anesthesia for delivery without adverse fetal effects. Hypotension is uncommon, but its incidence increases if the client doesn't receive a proper fluid load before the procedure. Epidural anesthesia may decrease the woman's urge to push.

Urgent cases
Spinal anesthesia involves an injection of medication into the cerebrospinal fluid in the spinal canal. Because of its rapid onset, spinal anesthesia is useful for urgent cesarean deliveries.

Delivery relief
Local infiltration involves an injection of anesthetic into the perineal nerves. It offers no relief from discomfort during labor but relieves pain during delivery.

Pain blocker I
A **pudendal block** involves blockage of the pudendal nerve. This procedure is used only for delivery.

Pain blocker II
A **paracervical block** involves the blockage of nerves in the peridural space at the sacral hiatus, which provides analgesia for the first and second stages of labor and anesthesia for delivery. This procedure increases the risk of forceps delivery.

Knockout drops
General anesthetics can be administered I.V. or through inhalation, resulting in unconsciousness. General anesthetics should be used only if regional anesthetics are contraindicated or in a rapidly developing emergency.

I.V. anesthetics, which are usually reserved for clients with massive blood loss, include ketamine (Ketalar).

Inhalation anesthetics include nitrous oxide and isoflurane (Forane).

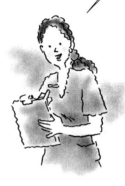

Hypotension after an epidural is uncommon but can occur if the client doesn't receive enough fluids beforehand.

Keep abreast of diagnostic tests

The key diagnostic test in the intrapartum period is fetal blood sampling.

Scratch the scalp
Fetal blood sampling is a method of monitoring fetal blood pH when indefinite or suspicious FHR patterns occur. The blood sample is usually taken from the scalp but may also be taken from the presenting part if the fetus

is in a breech presentation. Fetal blood sampling requires that:
- membranes be ruptured
- the cervix be dilated 2 to 3 cm
- the presenting part be no higher than −2 station.

A pH of 7.25 or higher is normal, 7.20 to 7.24 is preacidotic, and lower than 7.20 constitutes severe acidosis.

Nursing actions
- Explain the procedure to the client.
- After the procedure, observe the FHR and observe the client for vaginal bleeding, which may indicate fetal scalp bleeding.

Polish up on client care

Some potential intrapartum complications are abruptio placentae, amniotic fluid embolism, disseminated intravascular coagulation (DIC), dystocia, fetal distress, inverted uterus, laceration, precipitate labor, premature rupture of membranes (PROM), prolapsed umbilical cord, and uterine rupture.

Abruptio placentae

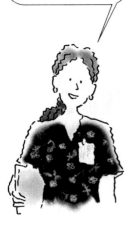

Abruptio placentae can occur anytime from 20 weeks' gestation through the second stage of labor.

Abruptio placentae refers to premature separation of the placenta from the uterine wall after 20 to 24 weeks of gestation. It may occur as late as the first or second stage of labor. Placental separation is measured by degree (from grades 0 to 3) to determine the fetal and maternal outcome.

Perinatal mortality depends on the degree of placental separation and fetal level of maturity. Most serious complications stem from hypoxia, prematurity, and anemia. The maternal mortality rate is about 6% and depends on the severity of bleeding, the presence of coagulation defects, hypofibrinogenemia, and the time lapse between placental separation and delivery.

CAUSES
- Abdominal trauma
- Cocaine or "crack" use
- Decreased blood flow to the placenta
- Hydramnios
- Multifetal pregnancy
- Other risk factors (low serum folic acid levels, vascular or renal disease, hypertensive disorders of pregnancy)

ASSESSMENT FINDINGS
- Acute abdominal pain
- Frequent, low-amplitude contractions (noted with an external fetal monitor)
- Hemorrhage, either concealed or apparent, with dark red vaginal bleeding
- Rigid abdomen
- Shock
- Uteroplacental insufficiency

DIAGNOSTIC TEST RESULTS
- Ultrasonography locates the placenta and may reveal a clot or hematoma.
- Coagulation studies may show evidence of DIC — increased partial thromboplastin time (PTT) and prothrombin time (PT), elevated level of fibrinogen degradation products, and decreased fibrinogen level.
- Hematology may reveal decreased platelet count if DIC is present.

NURSING DIAGNOSES
- Anxiety
- Deficient fluid volume
- Risk for decreased cardiac tissue perfusion

TREATMENT
- Transfusion: packed red blood cells (RBCs), platelets, and fresh frozen plasma, if necessary
- Cesarean birth

INTERVENTIONS AND RATIONALES
- Monitor maternal vital signs, FHR, uterine contractions, and vaginal bleeding *to assess maternal and fetal well-being.*
- Assess fluid and electrolyte balance *to assess renal function.*
- Avoid pelvic or vaginal examinations and enemas *to prevent further placental disruption.*
- Administer blood products and monitor vital signs *to detect adverse reactions.*

- Provide oxygen by mask *to minimize fetal hypoxia*.
- Position the client in a left lateral recumbent position *to help relieve pressure on the vena cava from an enlarged uterus, which could further compromise fetal circulation*.
- Provide emotional support *to allay client anxiety*.

Teaching topics
- Explanation of the disorder and treatment plan
- Activity restrictions

Amniotic fluid embolism

In amniotic fluid embolism, amniotic fluid escapes into the maternal circulation because of a defect in the membranes after rupture or partial abruptio placentae. During labor (or in the postpartum period), solid particles, such as skin cells, enter the maternal circulation and reach the lungs as small emboli, forcing a massive pulmonary embolism.

CAUSES
- Oxytocin (Pitocin) administration
- Abruptio placentae
- Polyhydramnios

ASSESSMENT FINDINGS
- Chest pain
- Hypertension
- Coughing with pink, frothy sputum
- Cyanosis
- Hemorrhage
- Increasing restlessness and anxiety
- Shock disproportionate to blood loss
- Sudden dyspnea
- Tachypnea
- Fetal bradycardia

DIAGNOSTIC TEST RESULTS
- Electronic fetal monitor reveals fetal distress (during the intrapartum period).
- Arterial blood gas (ABG) results reveal hypoxemia.
- Coagulation studies may reveal DIC.
- Chest X-ray reveals pulmonary edema.

NURSING DIAGNOSES
- Decreased cardiac output
- Impaired gas exchange
- Ineffective breathing pattern

TREATMENT
- Oxygen therapy: endotracheal intubation and mechanical ventilation if respiratory arrest occurs
- Cardiopulmonary resuscitation (CPR) if client is apneic and pulseless
- Continuous fetal monitoring
- Emergency delivery by cesarean birth
- Blood transfusion, if indicated
- Fluid replacement

Drug therapy
- Anticoagulant: heparin for DIC
- Vasopressor: dopamine
- Uterotonic: oxytocin (Pitocin)
- Activated factor VIIa for severe hemorrhage

INTERVENTIONS AND RATIONALES
- Monitor and record vital signs *to watch for tachycardia and tachypnea, which may indicate hypoxemia*.
- Assess respiratory and cardiovascular status *to detect early signs of compromise*.
- Assess FHR *to detect fetal distress*.
- Administer oxygen, as prescribed, *to improve oxygenation*.
- Assist with endotracheal intubation and mechanical ventilation, if necessary, *to maintain pulmonary function*.
- Perform CPR, if necessary, *to restore breathing and circulation*.
- Monitor and record intake and output *to detect deficient fluid volume*.
- Assist with immediate delivery of the neonate *to prevent fetal compromise*.

Teaching topics
- Explaining the disorder and treatment options to the client and her family

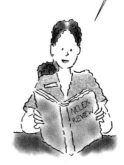

In amniotic fluid embolism, amniotic fluid escapes into the maternal circulation. It's an emergency that can require CPR.

Disseminated intravascular coagulation

DIC refers to increased production of pro-thrombin, platelets, and other coagulation factors, leading to widespread thrombus formation, depletion of clotting factors, and hemorrhage.

CAUSES
- Abruptio placentae
- Amniotic fluid embolism
- Retained fetus after demise

ASSESSMENT FINDINGS
- Abnormal bleeding (petechiae, hematomas, ecchymosis, cutaneous oozing)
- Nausea
- Oliguria
- Severe muscle, back, and abdominal pain
- Shock
- Vomiting

DIAGNOSTIC TEST RESULTS
- Coagulation studies reveal decreased fibrinogen level, positive D-dimer test specific for DIC, prolonged PT, and prolonged PTT.
- Hematology studies reveal decreased platelet count.

NURSING DIAGNOSES
- Risk for deficient fluid volume
- Ineffective tissue perfusion: Cardiopulmonary
- Decreased cardiac output

TREATMENT
- Transfusion therapy: packed RBCs, fresh frozen plasma, platelets, and cryoprecipitate
- Oxygen therapy
- Treatment of underlying condition
- Immediate delivery of the fetus by cesarean birth

Drug therapy
- Anticoagulant: heparin

Dystocia is long, difficult labor. It's experienced by about 10% of women during the first stage of labor.

INTERVENTIONS AND RATIONALES
- Monitor cardiovascular, respiratory, neurologic, GI, and renal status *to detect early signs of complications.*
- Monitor vital signs frequently *to detect signs of shock (increased tachycardia and hypotension).*
- Check all I.V. and venipuncture sites frequently for bleeding. Apply pressure to injection sites for at least 10 minutes. Alert other personnel to the client's tendency to hemorrhage. *These measures help to prevent hemorrhage.*
- Monitor intake and output *to detect signs of hypovolemia.*
- Enforce complete bed rest *to protect the client from injury.*
- Administer blood products and monitor the client closely for signs and symptoms of a transfusion reaction *to detect life-threatening complications.*
- Administer oxygen *to meet the body's increased oxygen demands.*
- Monitor the results of serial blood studies *to help guide the treatment plan.*

Teaching topics
- Explaining the disorder and treatment options to the client and her family
- Bleeding prevention

Dystocia

Dystocia is long, difficult, or abnormal labor. It's estimated that approximately 10% of women experience dystocia during the first stage of labor when the fetus assumes the vertex position.

CAUSES
- Problems with the power:
  - hypertonic uterine patterns
  - hypotonic uterine patterns
- Problems with the passenger:
  - fetal weight of 4500 g or more
  - malposition or malformation of the fetus
- Problems with the passage:
  - inadequate pelvic inlet

ASSESSMENT FINDINGS
- Arrested descent
- Hypertonic contractions
- Hypotonic contractions
- Prolonged active phase
- Prolonged deceleration phase
- Protracted latent phase
- Uncoordinated contractions

DIAGNOSTIC TEST RESULTS
- Ultrasonography shows fetal position or malformation or fetal weight greater than 4,500 g.
- Clinical pelvimetry identifies inadequate size of pelvic inlet.

NURSING DIAGNOSES
- Acute pain
- Deficient fluid volume
- Fear

TREATMENT
- Active management of labor
- I.V. fluid administration
- Delivery of the fetus by cesarean birth if labor fails to progress and the mother or fetus shows signs of compromise

Drug therapy
- Uterotonic: oxytocin (Pitocin) if contractions are ineffective

INTERVENTIONS AND RATIONALES
- Monitor maternal vital signs and FHR *to detect early signs of compromise.*
- Provide emotional support and encouragement *to help alleviate fear and anxiety.*
- Assist the client to a left side-lying position *to increase comfort and to relieve pressure on the vena cava from an enlarged uterus, which could compromise fetal circulation.*
- Encourage the client to void every 2 hours *to keep the bladder empty.*
- Monitor the effectiveness of oxytocin therapy and watch for complications *to ensure prompt intervention if complications occur.*

Teaching topics
- Explanation of the disorder and treatment plan

Fetal distress

Fetal distress refers to fetal compromise that results in a stressful and potentially lethal condition.

CAUSES
- Fetal hypoxia
- Prolapsed umbilical cord
- Unfavorable uterine environment
- Maternal causes: fever, drug use, illness
- Moderate to severe Rh factor isoimmunization

ASSESSMENT FINDINGS
- Meconium-stained fluid
- Electronic fetal monitoring reveals bradycardia or FHR greater than 180 beats/minute
- Maternal signs and symptoms of underlying illness
- Unsatisfactory progress of labor
- Loss of fetal movement

DIAGNOSTIC TEST RESULTS
- Fetal scalp blood sampling reveals acidosis.

NURSING DIAGNOSES
- Anxiety
- Fear
- Risk for decreased cardiac tissue perfusion

TREATMENT
- Supplemental oxygen by face mask, typically at 6 to 8 L/minute
- Amnioinfusion if the fetus exhibits variable deceleration not relieved by oxygen, positioning, or discontinuation of oxytocin (Pitocin) infusion (see *Understanding amnioinfusion*)
- I.V. fluid administration
- Emergency fetal delivery by vacuum aspiration, forceps, or cesarean birth

Drug therapy
- Discontinuing oxytocin infusion

INTERVENTIONS AND RATIONALES
- Monitor FHR, fetal activity, and fetal heart variability *to detect early signs of fetal compromise.*

Understanding amnioinfusion

Amnioinfusion is the replacement of amniotic fluid volume through intrauterine infusion of a saline solution, using a pressure catheter. This procedure is indicated for the treatment of repetitive variable decelerations not alleviated by maternal position change and oxygen administration.

Amnioinfusion relieves umbilical cord compression in such conditions as:
- oligohydramnios associated with postmaturity
- intrauterine growth retardation
- premature rupture of membranes.

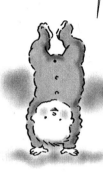

An inverted uterus can occur during delivery of the placenta.

• Monitor maternal vital signs and pulse oximetry *to detect early signs of compromise.*
• Notify the physician immediately of signs of compromise *to ensure prompt treatment.*
• Monitor intake and output *to detect early signs of deficient fluid volume.*
• Assist the client to a left side-lying position *to relieve pressure on the vena cava from an enlarged uterus, which could compromise fetal circulation.*

Teaching topics
• Explanation of the disorder and treatment plan

Inverted uterus

An inverted uterus can occur during delivery of the placenta. The inversion can be partial or total.

CAUSES
• Excessive cord traction
• Excessive fundal pressure

ASSESSMENT FINDINGS
• Large, sudden gush of blood from the vagina
• Signs of blood loss, such as hypotension, tachycardia, dizziness, paleness, and diaphoresis, which can progress to shock if blood loss continues unchecked for more than a few minutes
• Inability to palpate the fundus
• Severe uterine pain
• Uterine mass within the vaginal canal

DIAGNOSTIC TEST RESULTS
• Hematology tests reveal decreased levels of hemoglobin (Hb) and hematocrit (HCT).

NURSING DIAGNOSES
• Acute pain
• Deficient fluid volume
• Risk for decreased cardiac tissue perfusion

TREATMENT
• Fluid resuscitation with I.V. fluids and blood products
• Supplemental oxygen administration

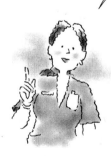

Here's a number to know: 500 ml or more of blood loss within 1 hour of delivery indicates postpartum hemorrhage.

• Immediate manual replacement of the uterus
• Possible emergency hysterectomy

Drug therapy
• Vasodilator: nitroglycerin to relax the uterus
• Tocolytic agent: terbutaline
• Oxytocic agent: oxytocin (Pitocin) after replacing the uterus to aid contraction
• Antibiotics to prevent infection because the uterus was exposed
• Analgesics: meperidine, morphine

INTERVENTIONS AND RATIONALES
• Administer supplemental oxygen *to meet increased oxygen demand.*
• Monitor vital signs frequently *to detect early signs of shock.*
• Monitor intake and output *to detect signs of deficient fluid volume.*
• Initiate CPR, if needed, *to restore circulation and breathing.*
• Assess the uterus for firmness, height, and position during the recovery phase *to detect complications.*
• Provide emotional support to the client and her family *to help allay fears and anxiety.*

Teaching topics
• Explanation of the disorder and treatment plan

Laceration

Laceration refers to tears in the perineum, vagina, or cervix from the stretching of tissues during delivery. Lacerations are classified as first, second, third, or fourth degree.

First-degree laceration involves the vaginal mucosa and the skin of the perineum and fourchette.

Second-degree laceration involves the vagina, perineal skin, fascia, levator ani muscle, and perineal body.

Third-degree laceration involves the entire perineum and the external anal sphincter.

Fourth-degree laceration involves the entire perineum and rectal sphincter and portions of the rectal mucosa.

CAUSES
- Large infant size
- Instruments used to facilitate birth
- Position of the fetus

ASSESSMENT FINDINGS
- Increased vaginal bleeding after delivery of placenta
- Evidence of laceration

DIAGNOSTIC TEST RESULTS
- Hematology studies may reveal decreased levels of Hb and HCT.

NURSING DIAGNOSES
- Acute pain
- Deficient fluid volume
- Fear

TREATMENT
- Laceration repair
- Cold application followed by heat application
- Sitz bath

Drug therapy
- Antibiotics possibly needed in some cases
- Analgesics: ibuprofen (Motrin), acetaminophen and oxycodone (Percocet), acetaminophen (Tylenol)
- Stool softener: docusate sodium (Colace)

INTERVENTIONS AND RATIONALES
- Monitor vital signs, including temperature, *to detect early signs of infection.*
- Monitor the laceration site for signs of infection and bleeding *to ensure prompt treatment interventions.*
- Insert an indwelling urinary catheter, if indicated, *to keep the perineal area clean and promote healing.*
- Provide maternal support and explain procedures *to allay anxiety.*

- Refrain from administering suppositories or enemas to a client with a third- or fourth-degree laceration *to prevent trauma to the repaired laceration site.*
- Apply cold packs to the perineal area for 12 hours, followed by heat packs and sitz baths for the next 12 hours, *to promote comfort and healing.*

Teaching topics
- Explanation of the disorder and treatment plan
- Perineal care
- Medication use and possible adverse effects

Precipitate labor

Precipitate labor occurs when uterine contractions are so strong that the woman delivers with only a few rapidly occurring contractions. It's commonly defined as labor completed within less than 3 hours. Such rapid labor may occur with multiparity. It may also follow induction of labor by oxytocin (Pitocin) or an amniotomy.

CAUSES
- Lack of maternal tissue resistance to the passage of the fetus
- Oxytocin administration
- Amniotomy

ASSESSMENT FINDINGS
- Cervical dilation greater than 5 cm/hour in a nulliparous woman; more than 10 cm/hour in a multiparous woman

DIAGNOSTIC TEST RESULTS
- There are no diagnostic test findings specific to this complication.

NURSING DIAGNOSES
- Anxiety
- Fear
- Risk for injury

TREATMENT
- Nonpharmacologic measures for pain control
- Controlled delivery to prevent maternal and fetal injury

Drug therapy
• Tocolytic agent: terbutaline to reduce the force and frequency of contractions

INTERVENTIONS AND RATIONALES
• Monitor FHR and variability *to detect early signs of fetal distress.*
• Monitor the infusion of a tocolytic drug *to detect early signs of adverse reactions.*
• Institute nonpharmacologic measures *to control pain, such as breathing exercises and distraction.*
• Provide emotional support *to allay anxiety and fear.*

Teaching topics
• Explanation of the disorder and treatment plan

Premature rupture of membranes

PROM is the rupture of membranes beyond 37 weeks' gestation but before the onset of labor. Chorioamnionitis may occur if the time between rupture of membranes and onset of labor is longer than 24 hours.

Preterm PROM is the rupture of membranes before 37 weeks' gestation.

CAUSES AND CONTRIBUTING FACTORS
• Cause unknown (however, malpresentation and a contracted pelvis commonly accompany the rupture)
• Lack of proper prenatal care
• Poor nutrition and hygiene
• Maternal smoking
• Incompetent cervix
• Increased uterine tension from hydramnios or multiple gestation
• Reduced amniotic membrane tensile strength
• Uterine infection

ASSESSMENT FINDINGS
• Fetal tachycardia
• Blood-tinged amniotic fluid gushing or leaking from the vagina
• Foul-smelling amniotic fluid if infection is present

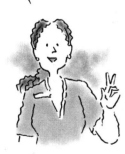

There are two types of PROM. Premature rupture occurs beyond 37 weeks' gestation but before the onset of labor. Preterm rupture occurs before 37 weeks' gestation.

• Maternal fever
• Uterine tenderness

DIAGNOSTIC TEST RESULTS
• Hematology studies may reveal an elevated white blood cell count if infection is present.
• Vaginal probe ultrasonography allows detection of an amniotic sac tear or rupture.
• Amniotic fluid culture and sensitivity identifies the causative organism of infection.

NURSING DIAGNOSES
• Anxiety
• Risk for infection
• Risk for injury

TREATMENT
• Hospitalization to monitor for maternal fever and leukocytosis and fetal tachycardia if the pregnancy is between 28 and 34 weeks (if infection is confirmed, labor must be induced)
• Cesarean birth if labor induction fails

Drug therapy
• Oxytocic agent: oxytocin (Pitocin) for labor induction if term pregnancy and labor doesn't result within 24 hours after membrane rupture
• Antibiotics according to culture and sensitivity results if infection is present

INTERVENTIONS AND RATIONALES
• Monitor for signs of labor and then progression of labor *to assess fetal progression.*
• Assess for signs of infection or fetal distress *to avoid treatment delay.*
• Administer antibiotics as prescribed *to treat infection and prevent complications.*
• Encourage the client to express her feelings and concerns *to allay her anxiety.*
• Monitor intake and output closely *to quickly identify signs of deficient fluid volume.*
• Assess the client for adverse reactions to oxytocin *to prevent complications.*

Teaching topics
• Explanation of the disorder and treatment plan

Prolapsed umbilical cord

A prolapsed umbilical cord occurs when the umbilical cord descends into the vagina before the presenting fetal part.

CAUSES
- Premature rupture of membranes
- Fetal presentation other than cephalic
- Placenta previa
- Intrauterine tumors that prevent the presenting part from engaging
- Small fetus
- Cephalopelvic disproportion that presents firm engagement
- Hydramnios
- Multiple gestation

ASSESSMENT FINDINGS
- Cord palpable during vaginal examination
- Cord visible at the vaginal opening
- Variable decelerations or bradycardia noted on the fetal monitor strip

DIAGNOSTIC TEST RESULTS
- Ultrasonography may reveal the cord as the presenting part.

NURSING DIAGNOSES
- Anxiety
- Risk for injury
- Risk for suffocation

TREATMENT
- Supplemental oxygen therapy at 10 L/ minute by face mask
- Maternal positioning on her hands and knees or with her hips elevated
- Immediate delivery of the fetus
- Nurse or physician maintaining a hand in the client's vagina until delivery occurs

Drug therapy
- Tocolytic agent: terbutaline may be used to reduce the force and frequency of contractions

INTERVENTIONS AND RATIONALES
- Place the client in Trendelenburg's position (position the woman's hips higher than her head in a knee-to-chest position) *to relieve pressure on the umbilical cord and restore blood flow to the fetus.*
- Administer supplemental oxygen *to help meet increased oxygen demands of the mother and fetus.*
- Apply warm saline-moistened towels to the protruding cord *to prevent drying and retard cooling of the cord.*
- Monitor FHR and variability *to detect early signs of fetal distress.*
- Assist with immediate delivery of the fetus *to prevent fetal death.*

Uterine rupture

Uterine rupture occurs when the uterus undergoes more strain than it can bear. Without emergency intervention, maternal and fetal death may occur.

CAUSES
- Prolonged labor
- Previous cesarean delivery
- Faulty presentation
- Multiple gestation
- Obstructed labor
- Uterine trauma

ASSESSMENT FINDINGS
- Abdominal pain and tenderness, especially at the peak of a contraction, or the feeling that "something ripped"
- Cessation of uterine contractions
- Chest pain or pain on inspiration
- Excessive external bleeding
- Hypovolemic shock caused by hemorrhage
- Late decelerations, reduced FHR variability, tachycardia and bradycardia, and cessation of FHR
- Palpation of the fetus outside the uterus
- Pathological retraction ring (indentation apparent across the abdomen and over the uterus)

DIAGNOSTIC TEST RESULTS
Diagnostic testing may not be possible in light of the life-threatening situation.
- Hematology tests reveal decreased levels of Hb and HCT.

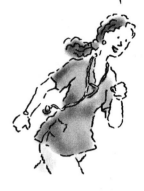

Umbilical cord prolapse is an emergency that requires prompt action to save the fetus.

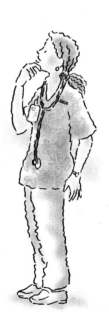

NURSING DIAGNOSES
- Acute pain
- Deficient fluid volume
- Ineffective tissue perfusion: Cardiopulmonary

TREATMENT
- Fluid resuscitation: I.V. fluids and blood products via rapid infusion
- Supplemental oxygen therapy, which may include endotracheal intubation and mechanical ventilation
- Surgery to remove the fetus and repair the tear, or hysterectomy, if necessary

Drug therapy
- Oxytocic agent: oxytocin (Pitocin) to help contract the uterus

INTERVENTIONS AND RATIONALES
- Monitor vital signs frequently *to detect signs of shock.*
- Prepare the client for immediate surgery *to avoid life-threatening treatment delay.*
- Administer supplemental oxygen *to meet increased oxygen demands.*
- Monitor I.V. fluid administration *to detect early signs of infiltration.*
- Monitor intake and output *to detect early signs of deficient fluid volume.*
- Assess cardiovascular, neurologic, and renal status *to detect early signs of compromise.*
- Provide emotional support to the parents *to promote healing in the occurrence of fetal demise or hysterectomy.*

Teaching topics
- Explanation of the disorder and treatment plan
- Postoperative care
- Availability of grief counseling

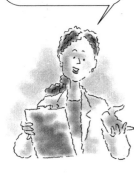

Note the most common complications requiring emergency birth: prolapsed umbilical cord, uterine rupture, and amniotic fluid embolism.

Emergency birth and preterm labor

Emergency birth and preterm labor are two examples of conditions requiring nursing care that may occur during the intrapartum period.

Emergency birth

Emergency delivery of the fetus may become necessary when the well-being of the mother or fetus is in jeopardy. Causes may include a prolapsed umbilical cord, uterine rupture, or amniotic fluid embolism.

CONTRIBUTING FACTORS
Contributing factors vary for each emergency birth situation.

Prolapsed umbilical cord
- Fetus presentation other than cephalic
- Hydramnios (excess of amniotic fluid)
- Multiple gestation
- Placenta previa
- Premature rupture of membranes

Uterine rupture
- Uterine trauma
- Previous uterine surgery
- Multiple gestation

Amniotic fluid embolism
- Abruptio placentae
- Polyhydramnios

ASSESSMENT FINDINGS
Data collection findings vary for each emergency birth situation.

Prolapsed umbilical cord
- Cord palpable during vaginal examination
- Cord visible at the vaginal opening
- Variable decelerations or bradycardia noted on the fetal monitor strip

Uterine rupture
- Abdominal pain and tenderness, especially at the peak of a contraction, or the feeling that "something ripped"
- Cessation of uterine contractions
- Chest pain or pain on inspiration
- Excessive external bleeding
- Hypovolemic shock caused by hemorrhage
- Late decelerations, reduced FHR variability, tachycardia and bradycardia, and cessation of FHR
- Palpation of the fetus outside the uterus

Amniotic fluid embolism
- Chest pain
- Coughing with pink, frothy sputum
- Cyanosis
- Hemorrhage
- Increasing restlessness and anxiety
- Shock disproportionate to blood loss
- Sudden dyspnea
- Tachypnea

DIAGNOSTIC TEST RESULTS
Prolapsed umbilical cord
- Ultrasonography confirms that the cord is prolapsed.

Uterine rupture
- Urinalysis can detect gross hematuria.
- Ultrasonography may reveal the absence of the amniotic cavity within the uterus.

Amniotic fluid embolism
- ABG analysis reveals hypoxemia.
- Hematology reveals thrombocytopenia, decreased fibrinogen level and platelet count, prolonged PT, and a PTT consistent with DIC.

NURSING DIAGNOSES
- Ineffective coping
- Acute pain
- Risk for infection

TREATMENT
- Administration of I.V. fluid
- Administration of oxygen by nasal cannula or mask (endotracheal intubation and mechanical ventilation may be necessary in the case of amniotic fluid embolism)
- Placing the client in left lateral recumbent position (for uterine rupture)
- Emergency hysterectomy (for uterine rupture)
- Emergency cesarean birth (see *Cesarean birth*)
- Possible transfusion of packed RBCs, fresh frozen plasma, or platelets

INTERVENTIONS AND RATIONALES
- Monitor maternal vital signs, pulse oximetry and intake and output as well as FHR *to assess for complications.*
- Administer maternal oxygen by cannula or mask at 8 to 10 L/minute *to maintain uteroplacental oxygenation.*

Management moments

Cesarean birth

Cesarean birth is the planned or emergency removal of the neonate from the uterus through an abdominal incision. A midline and vertical (classic) incision, allowing easy access to the fetus, is usually used in emergency situations. A low-segment, transverse, or Pfannenstiel (bikini) incision is usually chosen in a planned cesarean birth.

NURSING ACTIONS
- Provide emotional support and reassurance to the patient and her family, including reassurance about the well-being of the fetus.
- Assess fetal heart rate and maternal vital signs and intake and output.
- Monitor uterine contractions and labor progress, when appropriate.
- Obtain blood samples for hematocrit, hemoglobin level, prothrombin and partial thromboplastin times, fibrinogen level, platelet count, and typing and crossmatching.
- Maintain I.V. fluid replacement as necessary.
- Prepare the patient for surgery, including shaving of the abdomen and perineal area as necessary.
- Insert an indwelling urinary catheter as ordered.
- Provide preoperative teaching as necessary.
- Administer preoperative sedation as ordered.
- Provide immediate postoperative care.

> Therapeutic communication is key during emergency birth situations. The client and her family rely on you for support, reassurance, and information.

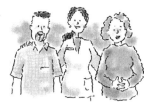

- Maintain I.V. fluid replacement *to replace volume loss.*
- Place the client in a left lateral recumbent position *to relieve pressure on the vena cava due to an enlarged uterus, which would compromise fetal circulation.*
- Provide emotional support and reassurance to the client *to allay fears and reduce anxiety.*
- Obtain blood samples to determine HCT, Hb level, PT and PTT, fibrinogen level, and platelet count and to type and crossmatch blood *to establish baseline values.*
- Monitor blood product administration, as necessary, *to replace volume loss.*
- Prepare the client and her family for the possibility of cesarean birth *to reduce anxiety.*

Teaching topics
- Reason for emergency birth
- Learning about procedures
- Understanding preoperative instruction
- Using breathing techniques

Preterm labor

Preterm labor, occurs before the end of the 37th week of gestation. Preterm labor can place both the mother and the fetus at high risk.

CAUSES AND CONTRIBUTING FACTORS
Causes of and contributing risk factors to preterm labor can be maternal or fetal.

> What can I say...sometimes I show up late, sometimes I show up early!

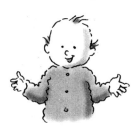

Maternal causes
- Abdominal surgery or trauma
- Cardiovascular and renal disease
- Dehydration
- Diabetes mellitus
- Incompetent cervix
- Infection
- Placental abnormalities
- Gestational hypertension
- PROM
- Smoking

Fetal causes
- Hydramnios
- Infection
- Multifetal pregnancy

ASSESSMENT FINDINGS
- Feeling of pelvic pressure or abdominal tightening
- Increased vaginal discharge
- Intestinal cramping
- Menstrual-like cramps
- Pain or discomfort in the vulva or thighs
- Persistent, low, dull backache
- Uterine contractions that result in cervical dilation and effacement
- Vaginal spotting

DIAGNOSTIC TEST RESULTS
- Electronic fetal monitoring confirms uterine contractions.
- Vaginal examination confirms cervical effacement and dilation.

NURSING DIAGNOSES
- Anxiety
- Deficient knowledge (treatment plan)
- Risk for injury

TREATMENT
- Suppression of preterm labor (if the fetal membranes are intact, there's no evidence of bleeding, the well-being of the fetus and mother isn't in jeopardy, cervical effacement is no more than 50%, and cervical dilation is less than 4 cm)
- Bed rest

Drug therapy
- Antibiotics according to organism sensitivity if urinary tract infection is present
- Betamethasone administered I.M. at regular intervals over 48 hours to increase fetal lung maturity in a fetus expected to be delivered preterm
- Nifedipine (Procardia), a calcium channel blocker, to decrease the production of calcium, a substance associated with the initiation of labor (adverse maternal effects include dizziness, nausea, bradycardia, and flushing)
- Indomethacin (Indocin) to decrease the production of prostaglandins and lipid compounds associated with the initiation of labor (adverse maternal effects include nausea, vomiting, and dyspepsia; premature closure of the fetus's ductus arteriosus can occur if indomethacin is given before 32 weeks' gestation)

- Magnesium sulfate to prevent a reflux of calcium into the myometrial cells, thereby maintaining a relaxed uterus
- Tocolytic agents, such as terbutaline and ritodrine (Yutopar), to inhibit uterine contractions (maternal adverse effects include tachycardia, hypoglycemia, hypokalemia, hypotension, and nervousness)

INTERVENTIONS AND RATIONALES

- Monitor maternal vital signs, contractions, and FHR every 15 minutes during tocolytic therapy (otherwise, provide continuous fetal monitoring) *to assess maternal and fetal well-being.*
- Notify the physician if the maternal pulse rate exceeds 120 beats/minute or the FHR exceeds 180 beats/minute *to expedite medical evaluation of maternal and fetal status.*
- Monitor the mother's respiratory status *to assess for pulmonary edema, an adverse effect associated with tocolytic therapy.*
- Monitor for maternal adverse reactions to terbutaline or ritodrine *to detect possible tachycardia, diarrhea, nervousness, tremors, nausea, vomiting, headache, hyperglycemia, hypoglycemia, hypokalemia, or pulmonary edema.*
- Provide emotional support to the mother *to ease anxiety and establish a therapeutic relationship.*
- Place the client in the lateral position *to increase placental perfusion.*
- Monitor for magnesium sulfate toxicity, which causes central nervous system depression in the mother and fetus, and make sure calcium gluconate is available *to reverse these effects.*
- Assess the neonate for possible adverse effects of indomethacin, such as premature closure of the ductus arteriosus.

Teaching topics

- Explanation of the disorder and treatment plan
- Medication use and possible adverse effects
- Following instructions for ongoing tocolytic therapy, if appropriate

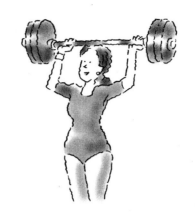

Pump up on practice questions

1. A client in the 28th week of gestation comes to the emergency department because she thinks that she's in labor. To confirm a diagnosis of preterm labor, the nurse would expect the physical examination to reveal:

1. irregular uterine contractions with no cervical dilation.
2. painful contractions with no cervical dilation.
3. regular uterine contractions with cervical dilation.
4. regular uterine contractions with no cervical dilation.

Answer: 3. Regular uterine contractions (every 10 minutes or more) along with cervical dilation before 36 weeks' gestation or rupture of fluids indicates preterm labor. Uterine contractions without cervical dilation don't indicate preterm labor.

➡ NCLEX keys

Client needs category: Physiological integrity
Client needs subcategory: Physiological adaptation
Cognitive level: Application

2. A client in the active phase of labor has a reactive fetal monitor strip and has been encouraged to walk. When she returns to bed for a monitor check, she complains of an urge to push. The nurse notes that the amniotic membranes have ruptured and that she can visualize the umbilical cord. What should the nurse do next?

1. Put the client in a knee-to-chest position.
2. Call the physician or midwife.
3. Push down on the uterine fundus.
4. Arrange for fetal blood sampling to assess for fetal acidosis.

Answer: 1. The knee-to-chest position decreases pressure on the baby and umbilical cord and improves blood flow. Calling the physician or midwife and arranging for blood sampling are important, but they have a lower priority than decreasing pressure on the cord. Pushing down on the fundus would increase the danger by further compromising blood flow.

➡ *NCLEX keys*
Client needs category: Physiological integrity
Client needs subcategory: Reduction of risk potential
Cognitive level: Analysis

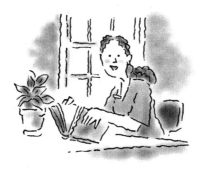

3. A client is attempting to deliver vaginally despite the fact that her previous delivery was by cesarean birth. Her contractions are 2 to 3 minutes apart, lasting from 75 to 100 seconds. Suddenly, the client complains of intense abdominal pain, and the fetal monitor stops picking up contractions. The nurse recognizes that which of the following has occurred?

1. Abruptio placentae
2. Prolapsed cord
3. Partial placenta previa
4. Complete uterine rupture

Answer: 4. In complete uterine rupture, the client would feel a sharp pain in the lower abdomen and contractions would cease. Fetal heart rate would also cease within a few minutes. Uterine irritability would continue to be indicated by the fetal heart monitor tracing with abruptio placentae. With a prolapsed cord, contractions would continue and there would be no pain from the prolapse itself. There would be vaginal bleeding with a partial placenta previa, but no pain outside of the expected pain of contractions.

➡ *NCLEX keys*
Client needs category: Physiological integrity
Client needs subcategory: Physiological adaptation
Cognitive level: Application

4. A client with gravida 3 para 2 (three pregnancies and two children) at 40 weeks' gestation is admitted with spontaneous contractions. The physician performs an amniotomy to augment her labor. The priority nursing action is to:

1. explain the rationale for the amniotomy to the client.
2. assess fetal heart tones after the amniotomy.
3. ambulate the client to strengthen the contraction pattern.
4. position the client in a lithotomy position to administer perineal care.

Answer: 2. The nurse should assess fetal heart tones after an amniotomy is performed because the umbilical cord may be washed down below the presenting part and cause umbilical cord compression. An explanation of the rationale for amniotomy would be given before the procedure. The nurse would ambulate the client only if the presenting part were engaged. Perineal care can be provided after assessing the fetal response to the amniotomy.

➡ *NCLEX keys*
Client needs category: Physiological integrity
Client needs subcategory: Reduction of risk potential
Cognitive level: Analysis

5. A nurse can consider the fetus's head to be engaged when:

1. the presenting part moves through the pelvis.
2. the fetal head rotates to pass through the ischial spines.

3. the fetal head extends as it passes under the symphysis pubis.
4. the biparietal diameter passes the pelvic inlet.

Answer: 4. The fetus's head is considered engaged when the biparietal diameter passes the pelvic inlet. The presenting part moving through the pelvis is called *descent.* Rotation of the head to pass through the ischial spines is called *internal rotation.* Extension of the head as it passes under the symphysis pubis is called *extension.*

➡ **NCLEX keys**
Client needs category: Health promotion and maintenance
Client needs subcategory: None
Cognitive level: Analysis

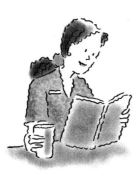

6. A client is dilated to 4 cm. She's asking for an epidural; however, her mother states that because of their culture, she has to "bite the bullet" as she did. What should the nurse do to make sure her client's request is honored?

1. Ask the client in a non-threatening way if it's her wish to have an epidural and then speak with the physician.
2. Honor the client's mother's request for no epidural.
3. Knowing the client's culture, have the family call a meeting to make the decision.
4. Call the anesthesiologist and request that he perform the epidural because the client is uncomfortable.

Answer: 1. It's up to the client to decide if she wants to have an epidural. The nurse is in the role of the advocate for the client. If a client is pregnant (at any age), she becomes emancipated and can make her own decisions. The client's mother or family can't override the client's decision. The nurse can't make the decision to call the physician without the client's consent. The nurse needs to clarify that the client does, in fact, want an epidural before contacting the anesthesiologist.

➡ **NCLEX keys**
Client needs category: Safe and effective care environment
Client needs subcategory: Management of care
Cognitive level: Analysis

7. The nurse receives orders for a client to receive a titrated infusion of oxytocin. Before starting the infusion, the nurse first:

1. initiates I.V. access.
2. checks the label on the infusion bag for proper concentration.
3. sets the infusion pump for the ordered rate.
4. identifies the client.

Answer: 4. The nurse must first identify the client because the infusion must be given to the correct client. Initiating I.V. access, checking the label on the infusion bag, and setting the infusion pump all address proper I.V. medication administration; however, the main concern is providing the infusion to the correct client.

➡ **NCLEX keys**
Client needs category: Safe and effective care environment
Client needs subcategory: Safety and infection control
Cognitive level: Application

8. A client in the second stage of labor experiences rupture of the membranes. The most appropriate intervention by the nurse is to:

1. assess the client's vital signs immediately.
2. observe for a prolapsed cord and monitor fetal heart rate (FHR).
3. administer oxygen through a face mask at 6 to 10 L/minute.
4. position the client on her left side.

Answer: 2. The nurse should immediately check for a prolapsed cord and monitor FHR. When the membranes rupture, the cord may become compressed between the fetus and the maternal cervix or pelvis, thus compromising fetoplacental perfusion. It isn't necessary to monitor maternal vital signs, administer oxygen, or position the client on her left side when the client's membranes rupture.

➡ **NCLEX keys**
Client needs category: Physiological integrity
Client needs subcategory: Reduction of risk potential
Cognitive level: Application

9. On the waveform, identify the area that indicates possible umbilical cord compression.

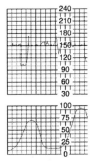

Answer: Variable decelerations are decreases in fetal heart rate that aren't related to the timing of contractions. Characteristic of umbilical cord compression, variable decelerations generally occur as drops of 10 to 60 beats/minute below the baseline.

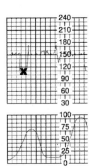

➡ **NCLEX keys**
Client needs category: Physiological integrity
Client needs subcategory: Reduction of risk potential
Cognitive level: Analysis

10. A client is receiving magnesium sulfate to help suppress preterm labor. The nurse should watch for which sign of magnesium toxicity?
   1. Headache
   2. Loss of deep tendon reflexes
   3. Palpitations
   4. Dyspepsia
Answer: 2. Magnesium toxicity causes signs of central nervous system depression, such as loss of deep tendon reflexes, paralysis, respiratory depression, drowsiness, lethargy, blurred vision, slurred speech, and confusion. Headache may be an adverse effect of calcium channel blockers, which are sometimes used to treat preterm labor. Palpitations are an adverse effect of terbutaline and ritodrine (Yutopar), which are also used to treat preterm labor. Dyspepsia may occur as an adverse effect of indomethacin (Indocin), a prostaglandin synthetase inhibitor used to suppress preterm labor.

➡ **NCLEX keys**
Client needs category: Physiological integrity
Client needs subcategory: Pharmacological and parenteral therapies
Cognitive level: Application

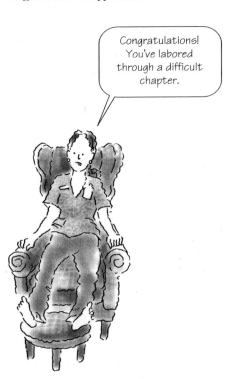

Congratulations! You've labored through a difficult chapter.

5 Postpartum care

In this chapter, you'll review:

✐ physiologic and psychological changes that occur immediately after pregnancy

✐ postpartum assessment

✐ how to care for postpartum complications.

Brush up on key concepts

A client undergoes both physiologic and psychological changes after delivery. Understanding these changes is essential to providing safe, effective client care.

At any time, you can review the major points of this chapter by consulting the *Cheat sheet* on page 74.

Physiologic changes after delivery

Here's a brief review of body system changes that occur immediately after delivery.

Circulation gyration
In the **vascular system,** blood volume decreases and hematocrit (HCT) increases after vaginal delivery. Excessive activation of blood-clotting factors also occurs. Blood volume returns to prenatal levels within 3 weeks.

Reproductive regeneration
In the **reproductive system,** uterine involution occurs rapidly immediately after delivery. Progesterone production ceases until the client's first ovulation. Endometrial regeneration begins after 6 weeks. The cervical opening is permanently altered from a circle to a jagged slit.

Hungry for hard work
GI system changes include:
• increased hunger after labor and delivery
• delayed bowel movement from decreased intestinal muscle tone and perineal discomfort
• increased thirst from fluids lost during labor and delivery.

Increasing capacity
Genitourinary system changes include:
• increased urine output during the first 24 to 72 hours after delivery due to an increased glomerular filtration rate and a drop in progesterone levels
• increased bladder capacity
• proteinuria caused by the catalytic process of involution (in 50% of women)
• decreased bladder-filling sensation caused by swollen and bruised tissues
• return of dilated ureters and renal pelvis to prepregnancy size after 6 weeks.

Hormone readjustment
In the **endocrine system,** thyroid function and the production of anterior pituitary gonadotropic hormones is increased. Simultaneously, the production of other hormones, including estrogen, aldosterone, progesterone, human chorionic gonadotropin, corticoids, and ketosteroids, decreases.

Psychological changes after pregnancy

More than 50% of women experience transient mood alterations immediately after pregnancy. This mood change is called **postpartum depression,** or the "baby blues," and signs and symptoms include sadness, crying, fatigue, and low self-esteem. Possible causes include hormonal changes, genetic predisposition, and adjustment to an altered role and self-concept.

Teach the client that mood swings and bouts of depression are normal postpartum responses; they typically occur during the

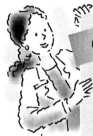

Cheat sheet

Postpartum care refresher

MASTITIS

Key signs and symptoms
- Chills
- Localized area of redness and inflammation on the breast with possible streaks over the breast
- Temperature of 101.1° F (38.4° C) or higher

Key test results
- Culture of purulent discharge may test positive for *Staphylococcus aureus*.

Key treatments
- Incision and drainage if abscess occurs
- Moist heat application to local area
- Pumping breasts to preserve breast-feeding ability if abscess occurs
- Analgesics: acetaminophen (Tylenol), ibuprofen (Advil)
- Antibiotics: cephalexin (Keflex), cefaclor (Raniclor), clindamycin (Cleocin)

Key interventions
- Administer antibiotic therapy.
- Apply moist heat.
- Encourage the client to breast-feed on the affected side before the unaffected side.

POSTPARTUM HEMORRHAGE

Key signs and symptoms
- Blood loss greater than 500 ml within a 24-hour period; may occur up to 6 weeks after delivery
- Signs of shock (tachycardia, hypotension, oliguria)
- Uterine atony

Key test results
- Hematology studies show decreased hemoglobin and hematocrit levels, a low fibrinogen level, and decreased partial thromboplastin time.

Key treatments
- Bimanual compression of the uterus and dilatation and curettage to remove clots
- I.V. replacement of fluids and blood
- Parenteral administration of methylergonovine (Methergine)
- Rapid I.V. infusion of dilute oxytocin (Pitocin)

Key interventions
- Massage the fundus and express clots from the uterus.

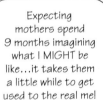

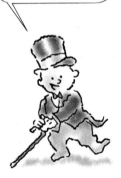

Expecting mothers spend 9 months imagining what I MIGHT be like...it takes them a little while to get used to the real me!

- Perform a pad count.
- Monitor the fundus for location.
- Monitor I.V. infusion of dilute oxytocin, as ordered.

PSYCHOLOGICAL MALADAPTATION

Key signs and symptoms
- Inability to stop crying
- Increased anxiety about self and neonate's health
- Overall feeling of sadness
- Unwillingness to be left alone

Key treatments
- Counseling for the client and family at risk
- Psychotherapy for the client
- Antidepressants: imipramine (Tofranil), nortriptyline (Pamelor)

Key interventions
- Obtain a health history during the antepartum period.
- Assess the client's support systems.
- Assess maternal-infant bonding.
- Provide emotional support and encouragement.

PUERPERAL INFECTION

Key signs and symptoms
- Abdominal pain and tenderness
- Purulent, foul-smelling lochia
- Tachycardia

Key test results
- Complete blood count may show an elevated white blood cell count in the upper ranges of normal (more than 30,000/µl) for the postpartum period.
- Cultures of the blood or the endocervical and uterine cavities may reveal the causative organism.

Key treatments
- Broad-spectrum I.V. antibiotic therapy, unless a causative organism is identified

Key interventions
- Monitor vital signs every 4 hours.
- Place the client in Fowler's position.
- Maintain I.V. fluid administration as ordered.
- Administer antibiotics as prescribed.

first 3 weeks after delivery and subside within 1 to 10 days.

Maternal behavior after delivery is divided into three phases:
- taking-in phase
- taking-hold phase
- letting-go phase.

What have I gotten myself into?

During the **taking-in phase** (1 to 2 days after delivery), the mother is passive and dependent, directing energy toward herself instead of toward her neonate. She may relive her labor and delivery experience to integrate the process into her life and may have difficulty making decisions.

Getting to know you

During the **taking-hold phase** (about 2 to 7 days after delivery), the mother has more energy and begins to act independently and initiate self-care activities. Although she may express a lack of confidence in her abilities, she accepts responsibility for her neonate and becomes receptive to neonate care and client teaching about self-care activities.

Assuming the role

During the **letting-go phase** (about 7 days after delivery), the mother begins to readjust to family members, assuming the mother role and the responsibility that comes with it. She relinquishes the neonate she has imagined during her pregnancy and accepts her real neonate as an entity separate from herself.

Keep abreast of postpartum assessment

The period immediately after labor and delivery is crucial to good postpartum nursing care. An understanding of normal and abnormal assessment findings is essential.

Monitor, monitor, monitor

The client's respiratory rate should return to normal after delivery. Other findings are listed below.
- The client's temperature may be elevated to 100.4° F (38° C) from dehydration and the exertion of labor.
- Blood pressure is usually normal within 24 hours of delivery.
- Bradycardia of 50 to 70 beats/minute is common during the first 6 to 10 days after delivery because of reductions in cardiac strain, stroke volume, and the vascular bed.

Nursing actions
- Monitor vital signs every 15 minutes for the first 1 to 2 hours, then every 4 hours for the first 24 hours, and then during every shift.

Fundal features

Check the tone and location of the **fundus** (the uppermost portion of the uterus) every 15 minutes for the first 1 to 2 hours after delivery and then during every shift. The involuting uterus should be at the midline. The fundus is usually:
- midway between the umbilicus and symphysis 1 to 2 hours after delivery
- 1 cm above or at the level of the umbilicus 12 hours after delivery
- 3 cm below the umbilicus by the third day after delivery
- firm to the touch.

The fundus will continue to descend about 1 cm/day until it isn't palpable above the symphysis (about 9 days after delivery). The uterus shrinks to its prepregnancy size 5 to 6 weeks after delivery.

A firm uterus helps control postpartum hemorrhage by clamping down on uterine blood vessels. The physician may prescribe oxytocin (Pitocin), ergonovine (Ergotrate), or methylergonovine (Methergine) to maintain uterine firmness. (See *Fundal assessment and massage,* page 76.)

Nursing actions
- Massage a boggy (soft) fundus gently; if the fundus doesn't become firm, use a stronger touch.

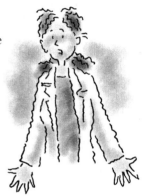

Studying for a big test can also cause mood swings—sometimes you may feel confident, other times anxious. Remind yourself that it's a normal reaction.

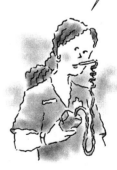

Clients commonly exhibit a slightly elevated temperature—up to 100.4° F—just after delivery.

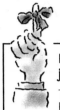

Memory jogger

To remember what to assess in the postpartum client, remember **BUBBLE**:

Breasts

Uterus

Bowels and bladder

Bonding

Lochia

Episiotomy.

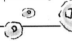

Fundal assessment and massage

WHY YOU DO IT
Fundal assessment is done to evaluate the progress of the uterus after birth, including uterine size, firmness, and descent. Fundal massage helps to maintain or stimulate uterine contractions, which are essential in preventing postpartum hemorrhage.

Assessment and massage should be performed every 15 minutes for the first hour after delivery, every 30 minutes for the next 2 hours, every hour for the next 4 hours, and then every 4 hours for the first postpartum day.

HOW YOU DO IT
• Explain the procedure to the client, and answer any questions. Provide privacy.
• Place the client in the supine position or with her head slightly elevated.
• Expose the abdomen and perineum.
• Gently compress the uterus between your hands to evaluate firmness and position in relation to the umbilicus (in fingerbreadths or centimeters).
• If the fundus seems soft and boggy, massage it gently in a circular motion until it's firm.
• Observe lochia flow during massage.
• Document the client's position, the firmness of the fundus, and the response to massage (if performed).

• Be aware that the uterus may relax if overstimulated by massage or medications.
• Suspect a distended bladder if the uterus isn't firm at the midline. A distended bladder can impede the downward descent of the uterus by pushing it upward and, possibly, to the side.
• Assess maternal-infant bonding by observing how the mother responds to her neonate.
• Assess for excessive vaginal bleeding.

Discharge diagnosis
Lochia is the discharge from the sloughing of the uterine decidua.
• **Lochia rubra** is the vaginal discharge that occurs for the first 2 to 3 days after delivery; it has a fleshy odor and is bloody with small clots.
• **Lochia serosa** refers to the vaginal discharge that occurs during days 3 through 9; it is pinkish or brown with a serosanguineous consistency and fleshy odor.
• **Lochia alba** is a yellow to white discharge that usually begins about 10 days after delivery; it may last from 2 to 6 weeks.

Some lochia characteristics may indicate the need for further intervention:
• Foul-smelling lochia may indicate an infection.

• Continuous seepage of bright red blood may indicate a cervical or vaginal laceration.
• Lochia that saturates a sanitary pad within 45 minutes usually indicates an abnormally heavy flow.
• Lochia may diminish after a cesarean birth.
• Numerous large clots should be evaluated further; they may interfere with involution.
• Lochia may be scant but should never be absent; absence may indicate postpartum infection.

Nursing actions
• Collect data on the color, amount, odor, and consistency of lochia every shift.

Breast check
Collect data on the size and shape of the client's **breasts** every shift, noting reddened areas, tenderness, and engorgement. Check the nipples for cracking, fissures, and soreness.

Nursing actions
• Advise the client to wear a support bra to maintain breast shape and enhance comfort.
• Tell the non-breast-feeding client that she can relieve discomfort from engorged breasts by wearing a support bra, applying ice packs, and taking prescribed medications.

Don't forget to communicate with my mother... she might have questions or might just need a little reassurance.

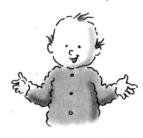

- If the client is breast-feeding, advise her that she can relieve breast engorgement by feeding the infant frequently, applying warm compresses, and expressing milk manually.
- Explain that nipples should be washed with plain water and allowed to air-dry. Soap and towel drying dries out nipples, causing cracking.

Elimination examination
Assess the client's **elimination** patterns. The client should void within the first 6 to 8 hours after delivery. If she doesn't, assess for a distended bladder, which can interfere with elimination and increase the risk of hemorrhage within the first few hours after delivery.

Nursing actions
- If the client can't urinate, pour warm water over the perineum to help stimulate voiding or insert a urinary catheter.
- Apply required ice packs or analgesic preparations to the client with hemorrhoids.
- Encourage the client to increase her fluid and fiber intake to prevent constipation.
- Administer laxatives, stool softeners, suppositories, or enemas as needed.
- Avoid rectal temperatures and enemas in clients who have a fourth-degree laceration.
- Alleviate maternal anxieties regarding pain from or damage to the episiotomy site.
- Encourage ambulation.

Evaluating episiotomy
The site of **episiotomy** (surgical incision into the perineum and vagina) should be assessed every shift to evaluate healing, noting erythema, intactness of stitches, edema, and any odor or drainage. Twenty-four hours after delivery, the edges of an episiotomy are usually sealed.

Nursing actions
- Administer medications to relieve discomfort from the episiotomy, uterine contractions, incisional pain, or engorged breasts as prescribed. Medications may include analgesics, stool softeners and laxatives, or oxytocic agents.

Teaching topics
- Explanation of the disorder and treatment plan
- Changing perineal pads frequently, removing from front to back
- Reporting lochia with a foul odor, heavy flow, or clots
- Showering daily to relieve discomfort of normal postpartum diaphoresis
- Following instructions on sexual activity and contraception
- Performing Kegel exercises to help strengthen the pubococcygeal muscles
- Sitting with the legs elevated for 30 minutes if lochia increases or lochia rubra returns, either of which may indicate excessive activity (notifying the physician if excessive vaginal discharge persists)
- Increasing protein and caloric intake to restore body tissues (if breast-feeding, increasing daily caloric intake by 200 kcal over the pregnancy requirement of 2,400 kcal)
- Relieving perineal discomfort from an episiotomy by using ice packs (for the first 8 to 12 hours to minimize edema); spray peri bottles; sitz baths; anesthetic sprays, creams, and pads; and prescribed pain medications

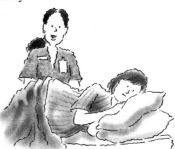

During assessment, position the client with a mediolateral episiotomy on her side to provide better visibility and prevent discomfort.

Polish up on client care

Potential postpartum complications include mastitis, postpartum hemorrhage, psychological maladaptation, and puerperal infection.

Mastitis

Mastitis is an infection of the lactating breast. It most commonly occurs during the second and third weeks after birth but can occur at any time.

CAUSES
- *Staphylococcus aureus* (the most common causative pathogen)

CONTRIBUTING FACTORS

*   Altered immune response
*   Constriction from a bra that's too tight (may interfere with complete emptying of the breast)
*   Engorgement and stasis of milk (usually precede mastitis)
*   Injury to the nipple, such as a crack or blister, which may allow causative organism to enter

ASSESSMENT FINDINGS

*   Aching muscles
*   Chills
*   Edema and breast heaviness
*   Fatigue
*   Headache
*   Localized area of redness and inflammation on the breast with possible streaks over the breast
*   Malaise
*   Purulent drainage
*   Temperature of 101.1° F (38.4° C) or higher

DIAGNOSTIC TEST RESULTS

*   Culture of the purulent discharge may test positive for the *S. aureus* bacteria.

NURSING DIAGNOSES

*   Ineffective coping
*   Acute pain
*   Situational low self-esteem

TREATMENT

*   Incision and drainage if abscess occurs
*   Moist heat application to local area
*   Pumping breasts to preserve breast-feeding ability if abscess occurs

Drug therapy

*   Analgesics: acetaminophen (Tylenol), ibuprofen (Advil)
*   Antibiotics: cephalexin (Keflex), cefaclor (Raniclor), clindamycin (Cleocin)

INTERVENTIONS AND RATIONALES

*   Monitor vital signs *to assess for complications.*
*   Administer antibiotic therapy *to treat infection.*
*   Apply moist heat *to increase circulation and reduce inflammation and edema.*

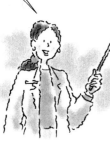

Uterine blood loss greater than 500 ml in a 24-hour period indicates postpartum hemorrhage.

*   Encourage the client to breast-feed on the affected side before the unaffected side *to promote complete emptying;* breast-feeding should be stopped and pumping initiated if an abscess occurs *to ensure emptying of the unaffected breast.*

Teaching topics

*   Positioning the infant during breast-feeding to avoid trauma to the nipples and milk stasis
*   Avoiding bras that are too tight and that may restrict the flow of milk
*   Breast-feeding every 2 to 3 hours and completely emptying the breasts
*   Changing nipple shields as soon as they become wet to prevent infection
*   Using a breast pump and discarding milk if breast abscess has developed

Postpartum hemorrhage

Postpartum hemorrhage is maternal blood loss from the uterus greater than 500 ml within a 24-hour period. It can occur immediately after delivery (within the first 24 hours) or later (during the remaining days of the 6-week puerperium).

CAUSES

*   Administration of magnesium sulfate
*   Cesarean birth
*   Clotting disorders
*   Disseminated intravascular coagulation
*   Forceps delivery
*   General anesthesia
*   Low implantation of placenta or placenta previa
*   Multiparity
*   Overdistention of uterus (multifetal pregnancy, hydramnios, large infant)
*   Perineal laceration
*   Precipitate labor or delivery
*   Previous postpartum hemorrhage
*   Previous uterine surgery
*   Prolonged labor
*   Retained placental fragments
*   Soft, boggy uterus, indicating relaxed uterine tone
*   Subinvolution of the uterus
*   Urinary bladder distention
*   Use of tocolytic drugs

ASSESSMENT FINDINGS
- Blood loss greater than 500 ml within a 24-hour period; may occur up to 6 weeks after delivery
- Perineal lacerations
- Retained placental fragments
- Signs of shock (tachycardia, hypotension, oliguria)
- Uterine atony

DIAGNOSTIC TEST RESULTS
- Hematology studies show decreased hemoglobin and HCT levels, a low fibrinogen level, and decreased partial thromboplastin time.

NURSING DIAGNOSES
- Ineffective peripheral tissue perfusion
- Deficient fluid volume
- Risk for infection

TREATMENT
- Bimanual compression of the uterus and dilatation and curettage to remove clots
- I.V. replacement of fluids and blood
- Abdominal hysterectomy if other interventions fail to control blood loss
- Urinary catheterization to empty the bladder

Drug therapy
- Parenteral administration of methylergonovine (Methergine)
- Rapid I.V. infusion of dilute oxytocin (Pitocin)

INTERVENTIONS AND RATIONALES
- Monitor vital signs *to assess for complications.*
- Massage the fundus and express clots from the uterus *to increase uterine contraction and tone.*
- Perform a pad count *to assess the amount of vaginal bleeding.*
- Monitor lochia, including amount, color, and odor, *to assess for infection.*
- Monitor the fundus for location *to assess for uterine displacement.*
- Monitor I.V. infusion of dilute oxytocin, as ordered, *to increase uterine contraction and tone.*
- Administer methylergonovine, as ordered, *to increase uterine contraction and tone.*
- Administer blood products and I.V. fluids, as prescribed, *to replace volume loss.*

- Provide emotional support *to help alleviate fears and anxiety.*
- Advise the client to request assistance with ambulation *to prevent injury.*

Teaching topics
- Explanation of the disorder and treatment plan
- Learning about surgical procedures, if appropriate
- Reporting changes in vaginal bleeding

Psychological maladaptation

Known as *postpartum depression,* psychological maladaptation is depression of a significant depth and duration after childbirth. Many postpartum clients experience some level of mood swings; psychological maladaptation refers to depression that lasts longer than 2 weeks, indicating a serious problem.

CAUSES AND CONTRIBUTING FACTORS
- Difficult pregnancy, labor, or delivery
- Neonatal complications
- History of depression
- Hormonal shifts as estrogen and progesterone levels decline
- Lack of support from family and friends
- Lack of self-esteem
- Stress in the home or work
- Troubled childhood

ASSESSMENT FINDINGS
- Extreme fatigue
- Inability to make decisions
- Inability to stop crying
- Increased anxiety about self and neonate's health
- Overall feeling of sadness
- Postpartum psychosis (hallucinations, delusions, potential for suicide or homicide)
- Psychosomatic symptoms (nausea, vomiting, diarrhea)
- Unwillingness to be left alone

DIAGNOSTIC TEST RESULTS
- There are no diagnostic test findings specific to this complication (diagnosis is based on signs and symptoms).

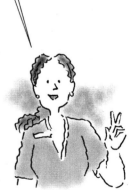

Although many clients experience some depression after childbirth, depression that lasts longer than 2 days should trigger your assessment alarm.

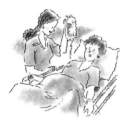

> Women who have undergone cesarean delivery are at higher risk for puerperal infection.

NURSING DIAGNOSES
- Fatigue
- Ineffective coping
- Social isolation

TREATMENT
- Counseling for the client and family at risk
- Group therapy
- Psychotherapy for the client

Drug therapy
- Antidepressants: imipramine (Tofranil), nortriptyline (Pamelor)

INTERVENTIONS AND RATIONALES
- Obtain a health history during the antepartum period *to assess whether the client is at risk for postpartum depression.*
- Assess the client's support systems *to determine the need for additional help.*
- Assess maternal-neonate bonding *to check for signs of depression.*
- Provide emotional support and encouragement *to reduce anxiety.*
- Notify a skilled professional if you observe psychotic symptoms in the client *to obtain necessary treatment.*

Teaching topics
- Explanation of the disorder and treatment plan
- Medication use and possible adverse effects
- Understanding that continued depression may require psychiatric counseling
- Understanding how to meet her own physical and emotional needs

> Placing the client in Fowler's position helps with the drainage of lochia.

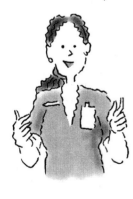

Puerperal infection

Puerperal infection occurs after childbirth in 2% to 5% of all women who have vaginal deliveries and in 15% to 20% of those who have cesarean births. Puerperal infection affects the uterus and structures above it and is one of the leading causes of maternal death.

CAUSES AND CONTRIBUTING FACTORS
- Bladder catheterization
- Cesarean birth
- Colonization of lower genital tract with pathogenic organisms, such as group B streptococci, *Chlamydia trachomatis*, *Staphylococcus aureus*, *Escherichia coli*, and *Gardnerella vaginalis*
- Episiotomy
- Forceps delivery
- Excessive number of vaginal examinations
- Intrauterine fetal monitoring
- Laceration
- History of previous infection
- Low socioeconomic status
- Medical conditions such as diabetes mellitus
- Poor general health
- Poor nutrition
- Prolonged labor
- Premature rupture of membranes
- Retained placental fragments
- Trauma

ASSESSMENT FINDINGS
- Abdominal pain and tenderness
- Anorexia
- Chills
- Fever
- Lethargy
- Malaise
- Purulent, foul-smelling lochia
- Subinvolution of the uterus
- Tachycardia
- Uterine cramping

DIAGNOSTIC TEST RESULTS
- Urine specimen may reveal the causative organism.
- Complete blood count may show an elevated white blood cell count in the upper ranges of normal (more than 30,000/µl) for the postpartum period.
- Cultures of the blood or of the endocervical and uterine cavities may reveal the causative organism.

NURSING DIAGNOSES
- Acute pain
- Risk for infection
- Social isolation

TREATMENT
- Administration of I.V. fluids (if hydration is needed)

Drug therapy
- Broad-spectrum I.V. antibiotic therapy, unless a causative organism is identified

INTERVENTIONS AND RATIONALES

- Monitor vital signs every 4 hours *to assess for complications.*
- Place the client in Fowler's position *to facilitate drainage of lochia.*
- Administer pain medication, as ordered, *to relieve pain and discomfort.*
- Provide emotional support and reassurance *to ease anxiety.*
- Maintain I.V. fluid administration, as ordered, *to replace volume loss.*
- Administer antibiotics, as prescribed, *to fight infection.*

Teaching topics

- Explanation of the disorder and treatment plan
- Medication use and possible adverse effects
- Recognizing signs and symptoms of a worsening condition, such as nausea, vomiting, absent bowel sounds, abdominal distention, and severe abdominal pain

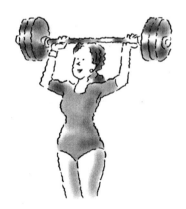

Pump up on practice questions

1.   When checking a postpartum client for uterine bleeding, the nurse finds the fundus to be boggy. After fundal massage by the nurse, the physician prescribes 0.2 mg of methylergonovine (Methergine) by mouth. What should the nurse tell the client?

1.   "Methergine is commonly used to help the uterus contract so that the bleeding will decrease. You may experience more cramping as your uterus becomes firmer."
2.   "You'll probably take this medication until you're discharged from the hospital. Every client usually needs to take this medication."
3.   "If your blood pressure is low, you won't be able to take this medication; I'll establish a new I.V. line so I can start Pitocin again."
4.   "Most people don't experience additional pain or cramping from taking this medication."

Answer: 1. Methylergonovine, an ergot alkaloid, is commonly given to stimulate sustained uterine contraction. It allows the uterus to remain contracted and firm, thus decreasing postpartum bleeding. Abdominal cramping, which may become painful, is a common adverse effect. Methylergonovine is discontinued when the lochia flow has decreased or the client complains of severe cramping. Clients may need only a few doses of methylergonovine to keep the uterus contracted. Methylergonovine is contraindicated in clients with high—not low—blood pressure.

➡ NCLEX keys

Client needs category: Physiological integrity
Client needs subcategory: Pharmacological and parenteral therapies
Cognitive level: Application

2.   A client had a cesarean birth and is postpartum day 1. She's asking for pain medication when the nurse enters the room to do her shift assessment. She states that her pain level is an 8 on a scale of 1 to 10. What should be the nurse's priority of care?

1.   Have the client get up to wash so that the bed can be made and the medication orders checked.
2.   Start the postpartum assessment.
3.   Check the orders for a pain medication and return for the assessment after the medication has relieved her discomfort.
4.   Tell the client to relax and the pain will subside.

Answer: 3. Pain management is a priority. Control of pain will enable the client to move, eliminating other potential complications of delivery. In addition, bonding with the infant will be facilitated if the client is without discomfort. The assessment should be initiated after pain management. Relaxation techniques will act as an adjunct therapy but isn't useful by itself for pain management during the postpartum period.

➡ NCLEX keys

Client needs category: Safe and effective care environment
Client needs subcategory: Management of care
Cognitive level: Analysis

3. A client delivered a neonate with spina bifida. She had been informed during the pregnancy that this was a potential risk. The nurse giving report states that this woman's decision to continue with the pregnancy was selfish, and now the neonate will suffer. In spite of the nurse's opinion, what ethical position should the nurse take when caring for this client and neonate?

1. Ask the client why she didn't have an abortion.
2. Accept the client's decision and care for the family as with any other patient.
3. Ask for another assignment because she doesn't agree with the decision the client made to continue the pregnancy.
4. Avoid going into the client's room if not necessary.

Answer: 2. It's the nurse's responsibility to care for and support the client and neonate. It isn't within the scope of care to judge a client or avoid responsibility.

➡ NCLEX keys

Client needs category: Safe and effective care environment
Client needs subcategory: Management of care
Cognitive level: Analysis

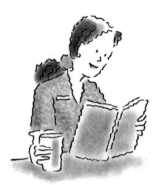

4. This is the client's first pregnancy. Her blood type is A– and her baby's blood type is A+. Before discharge, the client is scheduled to have a Rho(D) immune globulin (RhoGAM) vaccine. What's the most important action the nurse should take before administering the medication?

1. Ensure that the client understands and signs a consent form for the vaccination.
2. Choose a site for the injection that isn't tender.
3. Instruct the client that she won't need another vaccination after her next pregnancy.
4. Document that the injection was given in the chart.

Answer: 1. Before giving RhoGAM, the nurse needs to educate the client and make sure the client signs a consent form. Choosing a nontender site is not a priority. The client will need a subsequent vaccination after every pregnancy. Documentation is written in the chart after the injection is given.

➡ NCLEX keys

Client needs category: Safe and effective care environment
Client needs subcategory: Management of care
Cognitive Level: Application

5. During the third postpartum day, which finding is a nurse most likely to find in a client?

1. She's interested in learning more about neonate care.
2. She talks a lot about her birth experience.

3. She sleeps whenever the baby isn't present.
4. She requests help in choosing a name for the baby.

Answer: 1. The second to seventh days of postpartum care are the "taking-hold" phase, in which the new mother strives for independence and is eager for her baby. Talking about the birth experience, sleeping excessively, and asking for help in choosing a baby name describe the "taking-in phase," in which the mother relives her birth experience.

➡ *NCLEX keys*
Client needs category: Health promotion and maintenance
Client needs subcategory: None
Cognitive level: Analysis

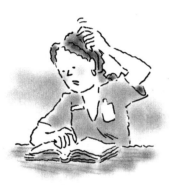

6. A client is 3 days postpartum. She states that she hasn't had a bowel movement since before delivery and is experiencing discomfort. She has had a fourth-degree laceration. The nurse knows that the best remedy is:
1. a suppository.
2. an enema to alleviate gas pains quickly.
3. stool softeners and fluids.
4. pain medication for the discomfort.

Answer: 3. A client with a fourth-degree laceration is at risk for dehiscence. Stool softeners and fluid will gently promote stool evacuation. Suppositories and an enema would be too harsh, and pain medications would slow down peristalsis of the intestines, slowing evacuation.

➡ *NCLEX keys*
Client needs category: Safe and effective environment
Client needs subcategory: Management of care
Cognitive level: Analysis

7. A nurse is providing care for a postpartum client. Which condition places this client at greater risk for a postpartum hemorrhage?
1. Hypertension
2. Uterine infection
3. Placenta previa
4. Severe pain

Answer: 3. A client with placenta previa is at greatest risk for postpartum hemorrhage. In placenta previa, the lower uterine segment doesn't contract as well as the fundal part of the uterus; therefore, more bleeding occurs. Hypertension, uterine infection, and severe pain don't place the client at increased risk for postpartum hemorrhage.

➡ *NCLEX keys*
Client needs category: Health promotion and maintenance
Client needs subcategory: None
Cognitive level: Analysis

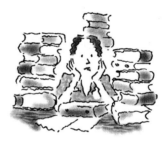

8. In performing a routine fundal assessment, a nurse finds that a client's fundus is boggy. What should the nurse do first?
1. Call the physician.
2. Massage the fundus.
3. Assess lochia flow.
4. Obtain an order for methylergonovine (Methergine).

Answer: 2. The nurse should begin to massage the uterus so that it will be stimulated to contract. Lochia flow can be assessed while the uterus is being massaged. The nurse shouldn't leave the client to call the physician. If the fundus remains boggy and the uterus continues to bleed, the nurse should use the call button to ask another nurse to call the physician. Methylergonovine may be prescribed, if needed.

➡ NCLEX keys

Client needs category: Physiological integrity
Client needs subcategory: Reduction of risk potential
Cognitive level: Application

9. Early discharge from the postpartum unit has safety issues that need to be discussed with the client during discharge education. What's the most important instruction that the nurse should give the new mom?

1. "Sleep when the neonate sleeps to avoid exhaustion."
2. "Don't sleep with the neonate in bed with you."
3. "If you have excessive vaginal bleeding, massage your fundus and call the physician."
4. "Don't worry; women have been having babies for years without postpartum problems."

Answer: 3. Excessive bleeding can lead to hemorrhage, causing the client to lose fluid balance and to faint. The client needs to massage her fundus and call the physician. While it's good advice to tell the client to sleep when the neonate sleeps, it isn't the most important instruction. Having the neonate sleep with the mother can be a potential hazard when rolling over causes suffocation; however, it isn't the most important instruction to give a client. Telling the client not to worry doesn't give her information about how to prevent a potentially life-threatening problem with postpartum hemorrhage.

➡ NCLEX keys

Client needs category: Safe and effective care environment
Clients needs subcategory: Management of care
Cognitive Level: Application

10. On a client's second postpartum visit, the physician reviews the chart note here regarding the client's lochia. What's the best term for the lochia described?

Flowsheet		
Lochia		
Date	10/12/10	10/13/10
Time	0945	0930
Color	Red	Red
Odor	Normal	Normal
Consistency	Few tiny clots	No clots
Amount	4 pads/ 24 hours	3 pads/ 24 hours

1. Alba
2. Thrombis
3. Rubra
4. Serosa

Answer: 3. Lochia rubra is a red discharge that occurs 1 to 3 days after birth. It consists almost entirely of blood with only small clots and mucus. Lochia alba is a creamy white or colorless discharge that occurs 10 to 14 days postpartum and may continue for up to 6 weeks. Lochia thrombis isn't a valid term. Lochia serosa is a pink or brownish discharge that occurs 4 to 10 days postpartum.

➡ NCLEX keys

Client needs category: Physiological integrity
Clients needs subcategory: Physiological adaptation
Cognitive level: Application

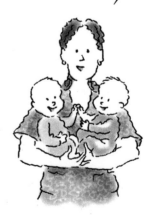

Just one more maternal-neonatal chapter to go. Let's do it!

6 Neonatal care

In this chapter, you'll review:

✐ neonatal adaptations to extrauterine life

✐ initial and ongoing neonatal assessment

✐ common neonatal disorders.

Brush up on key concepts

A neonate experiences many changes as he adapts to life outside the uterus. Knowledge of these changes and of the normal physiologic characteristics of the neonate provides the basis for normal neonatal care.

At any time, you can review the major points of this chapter by consulting the *Cheat sheet* on pages 86 and 87.

Adaptations to extrauterine life

Here's a review of how the neonate's body systems change.

Heart seals
The **cardiovascular system** changes from the very first breath, which expands the neonate's lungs and decreases pulmonary vascular resistance. Clamping the umbilical cord increases systemic vascular resistance and left atrial pressure, which functionally closes the foramen ovale (fibrosis may take from several weeks to a year).

Every breath you take
The **respiratory system** also begins to change with the first breath. The neonate's breathing is a reflex triggered in response to noise, light, and temperature and pressure changes. Air immediately replaces the fluid that filled the lungs before birth.

A delicate balance
Renal system function doesn't fully mature until between the second and third year of life; as a result, the neonate has a minimal range of chemical balance and safety. The neonate's limited ability to excrete drugs, coupled with excessive neonatal fluid loss, can rapidly lead to acidosis and fluid imbalances.

Digestive difficulties
The **GI system** also isn't fully developed because normal bacteria aren't present in the neonate's GI tract. The lower intestine contains meconium at birth; the first meconium (sterile, greenish black, and viscous) usually passes within 24 hours. Some aspects of GI development include:
• audible bowel sounds 1 hour after birth
• uncoordinated peristaltic activity in the esophagus for the first few days of life
• a limited ability to digest fats because amylase and lipase are absent at birth
• frequent regurgitation because of an immature cardiac sphincter.

Bun from the oven
Changes in neonatal **thermogenesis** depend on environment. In an optimal environment, the neonate can produce sufficient heat, but rapid heat loss may occur in a suboptimal thermal environment.

Disease control
The neonatal **immune system** depends largely on three immunoglobulins: immunoglobulin (Ig) G, IgM, and IgA. IgG (detected in the fetus at the third month of gestation) is a placentally transferred immunoglobulin, providing antibodies to bacterial and viral agents. The infant synthesizes its own IgG during the first 3 months of life, thus compensating for concurrent catabolism of maternal antibodies. By the 20th week of gestation, the fetus synthesizes IgM, which is undetectable at birth because it doesn't cross the placenta.

High levels of IgM in the neonate indicate a nonspecific infection. Secretory IgA (which

(Text continues on page 88.)

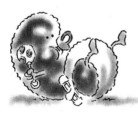

Because the renal system hasn't fully matured yet, the neonate can easily develop acidosis and fluid imbalances.

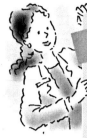

Cheat sheet

Neonatal care refresher

FETAL ALCOHOL SYNDROME
Key signs and symptoms
- Central nervous system dysfunction (decreased I.Q., developmental delays, neurologic abnormalities)
- Facial deformities
- Prenatal and postnatal growth retardation

Key test results
- Chest X-ray may reveal congenital heart defect.

Key treatments
- Swaddling
- I.V. phenobarbital

Key interventions
- Provide a stimulus-free environment for the neonate; darken the room, if necessary.
- Provide gavage feedings, if necessary.

HUMAN IMMUNODEFICIENCY VIRUS (HIV)
Key signs and symptoms
- Produces no symptoms (at birth)

Key test results
- Test interpretation is problematic because most neonates with an HIV-positive mother test positive at birth. Uninfected neonates lose this maternal antibody at 8 to 15 months, and infected neonates remain seropositive. Therefore, testing should be repeated at age 15 months.

Key treatments
- Antimicrobial therapy to treat opportunistic infections
- Zidovudine (Retrovir) recommended during the first 6 weeks of life based on the neonate's lymphocyte count

Key interventions
- Assess cardiovascular and respiratory status.
- Maintain standard precautions.
- Keep the umbilical stump meticulously clean.

HYPOTHERMIA
Key signs and symptoms
- Kicking and crying (a mechanism to increase the metabolic rate to produce body heat)

- Core body temperature lower than 97.7° F (36.5° C)

Key test results
- Arterial blood gas (ABG) analysis shows hypoxemia.
- Blood glucose level reveals hypoglycemia.

Key treatments
- Radiant warmer
- Skin-to-skin warmth (place neonate close to the mother)

Key interventions
- Dry the neonate immediately after delivery.
- Allow the mother to hold the neonate.
- Monitor vital signs every 15 to 30 minutes.
- Provide a knitted cap for the neonate.
- Place the neonate in a radiant warmer.

NEONATAL DRUG DEPENDENCY
Key signs and symptoms
- High-pitched cry
- Irritability
- Jitteriness
- Poor sleeping pattern
- Tremors

Key treatments
- Gavage feedings, if necessary
- Paregoric and phenobarbital to treat withdrawal symptoms; methadone shouldn't be given to neonates because of its addictive nature

Key interventions
- Monitor cardiovascular status.
- Use tight swaddling for comfort.
- Place the neonate in a dark, quiet environment.
- Encourage the use of a pacifier (in cases of heroin withdrawal).
- Be prepared to administer gavage feedings (in cases of methadone withdrawal).
- Maintain fluid and electrolyte balance.

Time for a change. I experience many bodily changes as I adapt to life outside the uterus.

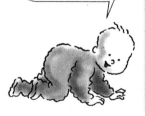

Neonatal care refresher *(continued)*

NEONATAL INFECTIONS

Key signs and symptoms
• Feeding pattern changes, such as poor sucking or decreased intake
• Sternal retractions
• Subtle, nonspecific behavioral changes, such as lethargy or hypotonia
• Temperature instability

Key test results
• Blood and urine cultures are positive for the causative organism, most commonly gram-positive beta-hemolytic streptococci and the gram-negative *Escherichia coli, Aerobacter, Proteus,* and *Klebsiella.*
• Complete blood count shows an increased white blood cell count.

Key treatments
• I.V. therapy to provide adequate hydration
• Antibiotic therapy: broad-spectrum until the causative organism is identified and then a specific antibiotic

Key interventions
• Assess cardiovascular and respiratory status.
• Administer broad-spectrum antibiotics before culture results are received and specific antibiotic therapy after results are received.

NEONATAL JAUNDICE

Key signs and symptoms
• Jaundice
• Lethargy

Key test results
• Bilirubin levels are elevated, with the rate of rise based on gestational age.

Key treatments
• Phototherapy (preferred treatment)
• Increased fluid intake

Key interventions
• Assess neurologic status.
• Monitor serum bilirubin levels.
• Initiate and maintain phototherapy (provide eye protection while under phototherapy lights and remove eye shields promptly when removed from the phototherapy lights).

RESPIRATORY DISTRESS SYNDROME

Key signs and symptoms
• Expiratory grunting
• Fine crackles and diminished breath sounds
• Seesaw respirations
• Sternal and substernal retractions
• Tachypnea (more than 60 breaths/minute)
• Tachycardia (more than 160 beats/minute)

Key test results
• ABG analysis reveals respiratory acidosis.
• Chest X-rays reveal bilateral diffuse reticulogranular density.

Key treatments
• Oxygen therapy with endotracheal intubation and mechanical ventilation
• Nutrition supplements (total parenteral nutrition [TPN] or enteral feedings, if possible)
• Surfactant replacement by way of endotracheal tube
• Temperature regulation with a radiant warmer

Key interventions
• Assess cardiovascular, respiratory, and neurologic status.
• Monitor vital signs and pulse oximetry readings.
• Initiate and maintain ventilatory support status.
• Administer medications, including endotracheal surfactant, as prescribed.
• Provide adequate nutrition through enteral feedings, if possible, or TPN.

TRACHEOESOPHAGEAL FISTULA

Key signs and symptoms
• Difficulty feeding, such as choking or aspiration; cyanosis during feeding
• Signs of respiratory distress (tachypnea, cyanosis, sternal and substernal retractions)

Key test results
• Abdominal X-ray shows the fistula and a gas-free abdomen.

Key treatments
• Emergency surgical intervention to prevent pneumonia, dehydration, and fluid and electrolyte imbalances
• Maintenance of a patent airway

Key interventions
• Assess cardiovascular, respiratory, and GI status.
• Place the neonate in high Fowler's position.
• Keep a laryngoscope and endotracheal tube at the bedside.
• Provide the neonate with a pacifier.
• Provide gastrostomy tube feedings postoperatively.

limits bacterial growth in the GI tract) is found in colostrum and breast milk.

Poietic license

In the neonatal **hematopoietic system,** blood volume accounts for 80 to 85 ml/kg of body weight. The neonate experiences prolonged coagulation time after birth because maternal stores of vitamin K become depleted and the neonate's immature liver can't produce enough to maintain adequate levels.

Nervous energy

The full-term neonate's **neurologic system** should produce equal strength and symmetry in responses and reflexes. Diminished or absent reflexes may indicate a serious neurologic problem, and asymmetrical responses may indicate trauma during birth, including nerve damage, paralysis, or fracture. Some neonatal reflexes gradually weaken and disappear during the early months.

Liver concerns

Increased serum levels of unconjugated bilirubin from increased red blood cell (RBC) lysis, altered bilirubin conjugation, or increased bilirubin reabsorption from the GI tract may cause jaundice — a major complication for the neonatal hepatic system. Physiologic jaundice appears after the first 24 hours of extrauterine life; pathologic jaundice is evident at birth or within the first 24 hours of extrauterine life; and breast milk jaundice appears after the 1st week of extrauterine life when physiologic jaundice is declining.

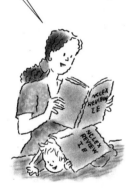

Physiologic jaundice is a mild jaundice that lasts for the first few days after birth.

Keep abreast of neonatal assessment

Neonatal assessment includes initial and ongoing assessments as well as a thorough physical examination.

First things first

Initial neonatal assessment involves detecting abnormalities and keeping accurate records.

Nursing actions

• Ensure a proper airway by suctioning, and administer oxygen as needed.
• Dry the neonate under a warmer while keeping the head lower than the trunk (to promote drainage of secretions).
• Apply a cord clamp, and monitor the neonate for abnormal bleeding from the cord; check the number of cord vessels.
• Observe the neonate for voiding and meconium; document the first void and stools.
• Check the neonate for gross abnormalities and clinical manifestations of suspected abnormalities.
• Continue to assess the neonate by using the Apgar score criteria even after the 5-minute score is received. (See *Apgar scoring.*)
• Obtain clear footprints and fingerprints (the neonate's footprints are kept on a record that includes the mother's fingerprints).
• Apply identification bands with matching numbers to the mother (one band) and neonate (two bands) before they leave the delivery room.
• Promote bonding between the mother and neonate.

Keep on keepin' on

Ongoing neonatal physical assessment includes observing and recording vital signs and administering prescribed medications.

Nursing actions

• Monitor the neonate's vital signs.
• Take the first temperature by the rectal route to determine whether the rectum is patent. Temperatures obtained by this route must be done gently to prevent injury to the rectal mucosa.
• Take the apical pulse for 60 seconds (normal rate is 120 to 160 beats/minute).
• Count respirations with a stethoscope for 60 seconds (normal rate is 30 to 60 breaths/ minute).
• Measure and record blood pressure (normal reading ranges from 60/40 mm Hg to 90/45 mm Hg).
• Measure and record the neonate's vital statistics (weight, length, and head and chest circumference).
• Complete a gestational age assessment.

Apgar scoring

The Apgar scoring system provides a way to evaluate the neonate's cardiopulmonary and neurologic status. The assessment is performed at 1 and 5 minutes after birth and repeated every 5 minutes until the infant stabilizes. A score of 8 to 10 indicates that the neonate is in no apparent distress; a score below 8 indicates that resuscitative measures may be needed.

Sign	0	1	2
Heart rate	Absent	Less than 100 beats/minute	Greater than 100 beats/minute
Respiratory effort	Absent	Slow, irregular	Good crying
Muscle tone	Flaccid	Some flexion of extremities	Active motion
Reflex irritability	None	Grimace	Vigorous cry
Color	Pale, blue	Body pink, blue extremities	Completely pink

• Administer prescribed medications such as vitamin K, which is a prophylactic against transient deficiency of coagulation factors II, VII, IX, and X.
• Administer erythromycin ointment, the drug of choice for neonatal eye prophylaxis, to prevent damage and blindness from conjunctivitis caused by *Neisseria gonorrhoeae* and *Chlamydia;* treatment is required by law.
• Administer the first hepatitis B vaccine within 12 hours after birth after obtaining parental consent.
• Perform laboratory tests.
• Monitor glucose levels and hematocrit (test results help assess for hypoglycemia and anemia).

Neonatal physical examination

The neonate should receive a thorough visual and physical examination of each body part. The following is a brief review of normal and abnormal neonatal physiology.

Heads up

The neonate's head is about one-fourth of its body size. The term **molding** refers to the shaping of the fetal head as it adapts to the shape of the birth canal. This is a normal occurrence with most births. The heads of most neonates return to their normal shape within 3 days after delivery.

Cranial complications that can occur include:
• cephalohematoma — blood collects between the skull and the periosteum; may occur on one or both sides of the head but doesn't cross the suture lines
• caput succedaneum — swelling in the soft tissues of the scalp, which can extend across the suture lines.

Closing time

The neonatal skull has two **fontanels:** a diamond-shaped anterior fontanel and a triangular-shaped posterior fontanel. The anterior fontanel is located at the juncture of the frontal and parietal bones, measures $1\frac{1}{8}$" to $1\frac{5}{8}$" (3 to 4 cm) long and $\frac{3}{4}$" to $1\frac{1}{8}$" (2 to 3 cm) wide, and closes in about 18 months. The posterior fontanel is located at the juncture of the occipital and parietal bones,

The heads of most neonates return to their normal shape within 3 days after delivery.

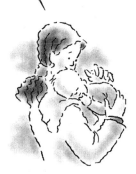

measures about ¾" across, and closes in 12 to 16 weeks. The fontanels:

- should feel soft to the touch
- shouldn't be depressed—a depressed fontanel may indicate dehydration
- shouldn't bulge—bulging fontanels require immediate attention because they may indicate increased intracranial pressure.

Jeepers peepers

- The neonate's eyes are usually blue or gray because of scleral thinness. Permanent eye color is established within 3 to 12 months.
- Lacrimal glands are immature at birth, resulting in tearless crying for up to 2 months.
- The neonate may demonstrate transient strabismus.
- Doll's eye reflex (when the head is rotated laterally, the eyes deviate in the opposite direction) may persist for about 10 days.
- Subconjunctival hemorrhages may appear from vascular tension changes during birth.

Nose only

Because infants are obligatory nose breathers for the first few months of life, nasal passages must be kept clear to ensure adequate respiration. Neonates instinctively sneeze to remove obstruction.

Dry mouth

The neonate's mouth usually has scant saliva and pink lips. Epstein's pearls (pearly, white, pinpoint papules) may be found on the gums or hard palate, and precocious teeth may also be apparent.

Sound check

The neonate's ears are characterized by incurving of the pinna and cartilage deposition. The top of the ear should be above or parallel to an imaginary line from the inner to the outer canthus of the eye. Low-set ears are associated with several syndromes, including chromosomal abnormalities.

The neonate should respond to sudden sounds by increasing his heart and respiratory rates.

For the neck of it

The neonate's neck is typically short and weak with deep folds of skin.

Flexi-chest

The neonatal chest is characterized by a cylindrical thorax and flexible ribs. Breast engorgement from maternal hormones may be apparent, and supernumerary nipples may be located below and medially to the true nipples.

Nice abs

The neonatal abdomen is usually cylindrical with some protrusion. A scaphoid appearance indicates diaphragmatic hernia. The umbilical cord is white and gelatinous with two arteries and one vein and begins to dry within 1 to 2 hours after delivery.

Teeny, tiny genitalia

Characteristics of a male neonate's genitalia include rugae on the scrotum and testes descended into the scrotum. The urinary meatus is located in one of three places:

- at the penile tip (normal)
- on the dorsal surface (epispadias)
- on the ventral surface (hypospadias).

In the female neonate, the labia majora cover the labia minora and clitoris, vaginal discharge from maternal hormones appears, and the hymenal tag is present.

Extreme measures

All neonates are bowlegged and have flat feet. Some neonates may have abnormal extremities. They may be polydactyl (more than five digits on an extremity) or syndactyl (two or more digits fused together).

Soldier straight

The neonatal spine should be straight and flat, and the anus should be patent without any fissure. Dimpling at the base of the spine is commonly associated with spina bifida.

Baby-smooth skin

The skin of a neonate can indicate many conditions—some quite normal and others

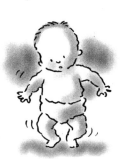

All neonates are bowlegged and have flat feet. Not to worry—most of us outgrow it.

requiring more serious attention. Assessment findings include:
• acrocyanosis (cyanosis of the hands and feet), which results from high levels of hemoglobin and vasomotor instability during the first week of life
• milia (clogged sebaceous glands) on the nose or chin
• lanugo (fine, downy hair) appearing after 20 weeks of gestation on the entire body except the palms and soles
• vernix caseosa (a white, cheesy protective coating composed of desquamated epithelial cells and sebum)
• erythema toxicum neonatorum (a transient, maculopapular rash)
• telangiectasia (flat, reddened vascular areas) appearing on the neck, upper eyelid, or upper lip
• port-wine stain (nevus flammeus), a capillary angioma located below the dermis and commonly found on the face
• strawberry hemangioma (nevus vasculosus), a capillary angioma located in the dermal and subdermal skin layers indicated by a rough, raised, sharply demarcated birthmark
• Mongolian spot, an area of bluish skin discoloration sometimes found in Blacks, Native Americans, and neonates of Mediterranean descent.

Reflections on reflexes

Normal neonates display a number of reflexes, which include:
• sucking: sucking motion begins when a nipple is placed in the neonate's mouth
• Moro's: when lifted above the crib and suddenly lowered, the arms and legs symmetrically extend and then abduct while the fingers spread to form a "C"
• rooting: when the cheek is stroked, the neonate turns his head in the direction of the stroke
• tonic neck (fencing position): when the neonate's head is turned while the neonate is lying supine, the extremities on the same side straighten while those on the opposite side flex
• Babinski's: when the sole on the side of the small toe is stroked, the neonate's toes fan upward
• palmar grasp: when a finger is placed in each of the neonate's hands, the neonate's

fingers grasp tightly enough to be pulled to a sitting position
• dancing or stepping: when held upright with the feet touching a flat surface, the neonate exhibits dancing or stepping movements
• startle: a loud noise, such as a hand clap, elicits neonatal arm abduction and elbow flexion; the neonate's hands stay clenched
• trunk incurvature: when a finger is run laterally down the neonate's spine, the trunk flexes and the pelvis swings toward the stimulated side.

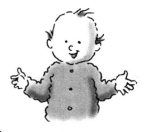

I have a repertoire of reflexes.

Polish up on client care

Potential neonatal complications and disorders include fetal alcohol syndrome (FAS), human immunodeficiency virus (HIV), hypothermia, drug dependency, infections, jaundice, respiratory distress syndrome, and tracheoesophageal fistula.

Fetal alcohol syndrome

FAS results from a mother's chronic or periodic intake of alcohol during pregnancy. The degree of alcohol consumption necessary to cause the syndrome varies. Because alcohol crosses the placenta in the same concentration as is present in the maternal bloodstream, alcohol consumption (particularly binge drinking) is especially dangerous during critical periods of organogenesis. The fetal liver isn't mature enough to detoxify alcohol.

CAUSES
• Risk of teratogenic effects increases proportionally with daily alcohol intake; FAS has been detected in neonates of even moderate drinkers (1 to 2 oz of alcohol daily)

ASSESSMENT FINDINGS
• Central nervous system dysfunction (decreased I.Q., developmental delays, neurologic abnormalities)

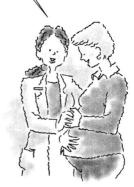

Warn mothers-to-be that binge drinking is even more detrimental than moderate daily alcohol consumption.

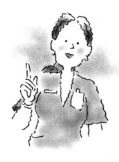

- Facial anomalies (microcephaly, microophthalmia, maxillary hypoplasia, short palpebral fissures)
- Prenatal and postnatal growth retardation
- Sleep disturbances (either always awake or always asleep, depending on the mother's alcohol level close to birth)
- Weak sucking reflex

DIAGNOSTIC TEST RESULTS
- Chest X-ray may reveal congenital heart defect.

NURSING DIAGNOSES
- Imbalanced nutrition: Less than body requirements
- Delayed growth and development
- Risk for impaired parenting

TREATMENT
- Swaddling

Drug therapy
- I.V. phenobarbital (to control hyperactivity and irritability)

INTERVENTIONS AND RATIONALES
- Provide a stimulus-free environment for the neonate; darken the room, if necessary, *to minimize stimuli.*
- Provide gavage feedings, as necessary, *to ensure adequate nutrition for the infant.*
- Refer the mother to an alcohol treatment center *for ongoing support and rehabilitation.*

Teaching topics
- Explanation of the disorder and treatment plan
- Expectations for the neonate's behavior
- Alcohol rehabilitation program

Human immunodeficiency virus

A mother can transmit HIV to her fetus transplacentally at various gestational ages — perinatally through maternal blood and bodily fluids and postnatally through breast milk. Administration of zidovudine to HIV-positive pregnant women significantly reduces the risk of transmission to the fetus.

CAUSES
- Transmission of the virus to the fetus or neonate from an HIV-positive mother

ASSESSMENT FINDINGS
- Produces no symptoms (at birth)
- Opportunistic infections (may appear by ages 3 to 6 months)

DIAGNOSTIC TEST RESULTS
- Test interpretation is problematic because most neonates with an HIV-positive mother test positive at birth. Uninfected neonates lose this maternal antibody at 8 to 15 months, and infected neonates remain seropositive. Therefore, testing should be repeated at age 15 months.
- HIV-deoxyribonucleic acid polymerase chain reaction or viral cultures for HIV should be performed at birth and again between ages 1 and 2 months.

NURSING DIAGNOSES
- Imbalanced nutrition: Less than body requirements
- Ineffective protection
- Risk for infection

TREATMENT
- I.V. fluid administration
- Nutritional supplements to prevent weight loss

Drug therapies
- Antimicrobial therapy to treat opportunistic infections
- Routine immunizations with killed viruses, except the varicella vaccines
- Zidovudine (Retrovir): recommended during the first 6 weeks of life based on the neonate's lymphocyte count to prevent perinatal transmission.
- Combination therapy: recommended when HIV infection is confirmed; therapy should include zidovudine combined with lamivudine (Epivir) or didanosine (Videx); or lamivudine combined with didanosine

INTERVENTIONS AND RATIONALES
- Assess the neonate's cardiovascular and respiratory status *for complications.*
- Monitor vital signs and fluid intake and output *to assess for dehydration.*
- Monitor fluid and electrolyte status *to guide fluid and electrolyte replacement therapy.*
- Keep the umbilical stump meticulously clean *to prevent opportunistic infection.*
- Maintain standard precautions *to prevent the spread of infection.*
- Administer medications, as indicated, *to treat infection and improve immune function.*
- Provide emotional support to the family *to allay anxiety*
- Monitor the neonate for signs of opportunistic infection *to prevent treatment delay.*

Teaching topics
- Explanation of the disorder and treatment plan
- Medication use and possible adverse effects
- Avoiding infection
- Importance of nutrition
- Providing the child with all necessary immunizations

Hypothermia

A neonate's temperature is about 99° F (37.2° C) at birth. Inside the womb, the fetus was confined in an environment where the temperature was constant. At birth, this temperature can fall rapidly.

CAUSES
- Cold temperature in delivery environment
- Heat loss due to evaporation, conduction, radiation, or convection
- Immature temperature-regulating system
- Inability to conserve heat because of little subcutaneous fat (brown fat store)

ASSESSMENT FINDINGS
- Kicking and crying (a mechanism to increase the metabolic rate to produce body heat)
- Core body temperature lower than 97.7° F (36.5° C)
- Lethargy with extreme hypothermia

DIAGNOSTIC TEST RESULTS
- Arterial blood gas (ABG) analysis shows hypoxemia.
- Blood glucose level reveals hypoglycemia.

NURSING DIAGNOSES
- Hypothermia
- Ineffective thermoregulation
- Risk for impaired parenting

TREATMENT
- Radiant warmer
- Skin-to-skin warmth (place the neonate close to the mother)

INTERVENTIONS AND RATIONALES
- Dry the neonate immediately after delivery *to prevent heat loss.*
- Wrap the neonate in a warm blanket *to help stabilize body temperature.*
- Allow the mother to hold the neonate *to provide warmth.*
- Monitor vital signs every 15 to 30 minutes *to assess temperature fluctuations and complications.*
- Provide a knitted cap for the neonate *to prevent heat loss through the head.*
- Place the neonate in a radiant warmer *to maintain thermoregulation.*

Teaching topics
- Preventing hypothermia
- Stressing infant-parent bonding (see *Teaching neonatal care to parents,* page 94)

Neonatal drug dependency

Neonates born to drug-addicted mothers are at risk for preterm birth, aspiration pneumonia, meconium-stained fluid, and meconium aspiration. Drug-dependent neonates also may experience withdrawal from such substances as heroin and cocaine.

CAUSES
- Drug addiction in the mother

ASSESSMENT FINDINGS
- Diarrhea
- Frequent sneezing and yawning

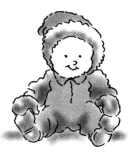

Brrr... In the womb, the temperature was constant. At birth, my temperature may fall rapidly.

Teaching neonatal care to parents

Here are some topics to include when teaching parents about caring for their neonate.

CORD CARE

With every diaper change, wipe the umbilical cord with water, especially around the base. Report any odor, discharge, or signs of skin irritation around the cord. Fold the diaper below the cord until the cord falls off, usually in 1 to 2 weeks.

CIRCUMCISION CARE

Gently clean the circumcised penis with water, and apply fresh petroleum gauze with each diaper change. Loosen the petroleum gauze stuck to the penis by pouring warm water over the area. Don't remove yellow discharge that covers the glans after circumcision; this is part of normal healing. Report any foul-smelling, purulent discharge promptly. Apply diapers loosely until the circumcision heals after about 5 days.

If the plastibell method of circumcision was used, leave the plastic ring in place until it falls off on its own, typically in 5 to 8 days. No special dressing is applied, and bathing and diapering are performed normally.

UNCIRCUMCISED CARE

Don't retract the foreskin when washing the uncircumcised penis because the foreskin is adhered to the glans.

POTTY PATTERNS

Become familiar with the neonate's voiding and elimination patterns:

• The neonate's first stools are called *meconium;* they are odorless, dark green, and thick.
• Transitional stools occur about 2 to 3 days after the ingestion of milk; they're greenish brown and thinner than meconium.
• The stools change to pasty yellow and pungent (bottle-fed neonate) or loose yellow and sweet-smelling (breast-fed neonate) by the fourth day.
• Change diapers before and after every feeding; expose the neonate's buttocks to the air and light several times a day for about 20 minutes to treat diaper rash.

BATH TIME

Give the neonate sponge baths until the cord falls off; then wash the neonate in a tub containing 3" to 4" (7.5 to 10 cm) of warm water.

MEALTIME AT THE BREAST

Initiate breast-feeding as soon as possible after delivery, and then feed the neonate on demand. Follow these guidelines:
• Position the neonate's mouth slightly differently at each feeding to reduce irritation at one site.
• Burp the neonate before switching to the other breast.
• Insert the little finger into a corner of the neonate's mouth to separate the neonate from the nipple.
• Experiment with various breast-feeding positions.
• Perform thorough breast care to promote cleanliness and comfort.

• Follow a diet that ensures adequate nutrition for the mother and neonate (drink at least four 8-oz glasses of fluid daily, increase caloric intake by 200 kcal over the pregnancy requirement of 2,400 kcal, avoid foods that cause irritability, gas, or diarrhea).
• Consult the physician before taking any medication.
• Know that ingested substances (caffeine, alcohol, and medications) can pass into breast milk.

MEALTIME WITH THE BOTTLE

Follow the pediatrician's instructions for preparing and feeding with formula. Follow these guidelines:
• Feed the neonate in an upright position, and keep the nipple full of formula to minimize air swallowing.
• Burp the neonate after each ounce of formula or more frequently if the neonate spits up.

SAFETY SEATS

Make sure parents understand the importance of using child safety seats. Instruct them to place the neonate in the back seat facing to the rear until the neonate is over 20 lb (9 kg) and older than 1 year. Stress the proper use of car seats by following the manufacturer's recommendations for placement and weight.

• High-pitched cry
• Hyperactive reflexes
• Increased tendon reflexes
• Irritability
• Jitteriness
• Poor feeding habits

• Poor sleeping pattern
• Tremors
• Inability to be consoled
• Vigorous sucking on hands
• Withdrawal symptoms (depend on the length of maternal addiction, the drug

ingested, and the time of last ingestion before delivery; usually appear within 24 hours of delivery)

DIAGNOSTIC TEST RESULTS
- Drug screen reveals agent abused by the mother.

NURSING DIAGNOSES
- Imbalanced nutrition: Less than body requirements.
- Risk for imbalanced fluid volume
- Risk for injury

TREATMENT
- Gavage feedings, if necessary
- I.V. therapy to maintain hydration

Drug therapy
- Paregoric and phenobarbital to treat withdrawal symptoms (methadone shouldn't be given to neonates because of its addictive nature)

INTERVENTIONS AND RATIONALES
- Monitor cardiovascular status *to detect cardiovascular compromise.*
- Monitor vital signs and fluid intake and output *to assess for complications.*
- Encourage the mother to hold the neonate *to promote maternal-infant bonding.*
- Use tight swaddling *for comfort.*
- Place the neonate in a dark, quiet room *to provide a stimulus-free environment.*
- Encourage the use of a pacifier *to meet sucking needs* (in cases of heroin withdrawal).
- Be prepared to administer gavage feedings *because of the neonate's poor sucking reflex* (in cases of methadone withdrawal).
- Maintain fluid and electrolyte balance *to replace fluid loss.*
- Monitor bilirubin levels and assess for jaundice (in cases of methadone withdrawal) *to assess for liver damage.*

Teaching topics
- Explanation of the disorder and treatment plan
- Expectations for the neonate's behavior
- Importance of nutrition
- Avoiding breast-feeding

Neonatal infections

A neonate may contract an infection before, during, or after delivery. Maternal IgM doesn't cross the placenta, and IgA requires time to reach optimum levels after birth, limiting the neonate's immune response. Dysmaturity caused by intrauterine growth retardation, preterm birth, or postterm birth can further compromise the neonate's immune system and predispose him to infection.

Sepsis is one of the most significant causes of neonatal morbidity and mortality. Toxoplasmosis, syphilis, rubella, cytomegalovirus, and herpes are common perinatal infections known to affect neonates. Beta-hemolytic streptococci infection may occur as a result of contact with the maternal genital tract during labor and delivery.

CAUSES
- Chorioamnionitis
- Low birth weight or premature birth
- Maternal substance abuse
- Maternal urinary tract infections
- Meconium aspiration
- Nosocomial infection
- Premature labor
- Prolonged maternal rupture of membranes

ASSESSMENT FINDINGS
- Abdominal distention
- Apnea
- Feeding pattern changes, such as poor sucking or decreased intake
- Hyperbilirubinemia
- Pallor
- Petechiae
- Poor weight gain
- Sternal retractions
- Subtle, nonspecific behavioral changes, such as lethargy or hypotonia
- Tachycardia
- Temperature instability
- Vomiting
- Diarrhea

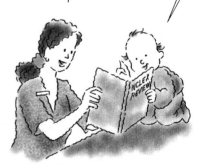

There's a lot to know about neonatal care... how did we get ourselves into this, anyway?

What do you mean "we"? I'm not taking the NCLEX!

DIAGNOSTIC TEST RESULTS

- Blood and urine cultures are positive for the causative organism, most commonly gram-positive beta-hemolytic streptococci and the gram-negative *Escherichia coli, Aerobacter, Proteus,* and *Klebsiella.*
- Blood chemistry shows increased direct bilirubin levels.
- Complete blood count shows an increased white blood cell count.
- Lumbar puncture is positive for causative organisms.

NURSING DIAGNOSES

- Imbalanced nutrition: Less than body requirements
- Hypothermia
- Risk for imbalanced fluid volume

TREATMENT

- Gastric aspiration
- I.V. therapy to provide adequate hydration

Drug therapy

- Antibiotic therapy: broad-spectrum until the causative organism is identified and then a specific antibiotic

INTERVENTIONS AND RATIONALES

- Assess cardiovascular and respiratory status *for complications.*
- Monitor vital signs *to assess for complications.*
- Monitor fluid and electrolyte status *to assess the need for fluid replacement.*
- Initiate and maintain respiratory support, as needed, *to maintain respiratory filtration.*
- Administer broad-spectrum antibiotics before culture results are received, and specific antibiotic therapy after results are received, *to treat infection.*
- Provide the family with reassurance and support *to reduce anxiety.*
- Provide the neonate with physiologic supportive care *to maintain a neutral thermal environment.*
- Maintain I.V. therapy, as ordered, *to replace fluid loss.*
- Obtain blood samples and urine specimens *to assess antibiotic therapy efficacy.*

Teaching topics

- Explanation of the disorder and treatment plan
- Knowing the importance of continuing drug therapy for the duration prescribed
- Preventing infection

Neonatal jaundice

Also called *hyperbilirubinemia,* neonatal jaundice is characterized by a bilirubin level that:

- exceeds 6 mg/dl within the first 24 hours after delivery
- remains elevated beyond 7 days (in a full-term neonate)
- remains elevated for 10 days (in a premature neonate).

The neonate's bilirubin levels rise as bilirubin production exceeds the liver's capacity to metabolize it. Unbound, unconjugated bilirubin can easily cross the blood-brain barrier, leading to kernicterus (an encephalopathy).

CAUSES

- Absence of intestinal flora needed for bilirubin passage in the bowel
- Enclosed hemorrhage
- Erythroblastosis fetalis (hemolytic disease of the neonate)
- Hypoglycemia
- Hypothermia
- Impaired hepatic functioning
- Neonatal asphyxia (respiratory failure in the neonate)
- Polycythemia
- Prematurity
- Reduced bowel motility and delayed meconium passage
- Sepsis

ASSESSMENT FINDINGS

- Jaundice
- Lethargy
- Decreased reflexes
- High-pitched crying
- Opisthotonos
- Seizures

DIAGNOSTIC TEST RESULTS
• Bilirubin levels are elevated, with the rate of rise based on gestational age.
• Conjugated (direct) bilirubin levels exceed 2 mg/dl.
• Bilirubin levels rise by more than 5 mg/day.

NURSING DIAGNOSES
• Impaired parenting
• Deficient fluid volume
• Risk for injury

TREATMENT
• Phototherapy (preferred treatment)
• Exchange transfusion to remove maternal antibodies and sensitized RBCs if phototherapy fails
• Increased fluid intake
• Treatment for anemia if jaundice is caused by hemolytic disease

INTERVENTIONS AND RATIONALES
• Assess neurologic status *for signs of encephalopathy, which indicates the potential for permanent damage.*
• Maintain a neutral thermal environment *to prevent hypothermia.*
• Monitor serum bilirubin levels *to assess for increased or decreased levels of bilirubin.*
• Initiate and maintain phototherapy (provide eye protection while the neonate is under phototherapy lights, and remove eye shields promptly when he's removed from the phototherapy lights) *to prevent complications.*
• Allow time for maternal-neonate bonding and interaction during phototherapy *to promote bonding.*
• Keep the neonate's anal area clean and dry. *Frequent, greenish stools result from bilirubin excretion and can lead to skin irritations.*
• Provide the parents with support, reassurance, and encouragement *to reduce anxiety.*

Teaching topics
• Explanation of the disorder and treatment plan
• Encouraging frequent feedings to maintain adequate caloric intake and hydration and to facilitate excretion of waste

Respiratory distress syndrome

Respiratory distress syndrome occurs most commonly in preterm neonates of diabetic mothers and neonates delivered by cesarean births. In respiratory distress syndrome, a hyaline-like membrane lines the terminal bronchioles, alveolar ducts, and alveoli, preventing exchange of oxygen and carbon dioxide.

CAUSES
• Inability to maintain alveolar stability
• Low level or absence of surfactant

ASSESSMENT FINDINGS
• Cyanosis
• Expiratory grunting
• Fine crackles and diminished breath sounds
• Hypothermia
• Nasal flaring
• Respiratory acidosis
• Seesaw respirations
• Sternal and substernal retractions
• Tachypnea (more than 60 breaths/minute)
• Tachycardia (more than 160 beats/minute)

DIAGNOSTIC TEST RESULTS
• ABG analysis reveals respiratory acidosis.
• Chest X-rays reveal bilateral diffuse reticulogranular density.

NURSING DIAGNOSES
• Imbalanced nutrition: Less than body requirements
• Ineffective tissue perfusion: Cardiopulmonary
• Impaired gas exchange

TREATMENT
• Acid-base balance maintenance
• Oxygen therapy with endotracheal intubation and mechanical ventilation
• Nutrition supplements (total parenteral nutrition [TPN] or enteral feedings, if possible)
• Surfactant replacement by way of endotracheal tube
• Temperature regulation with a radiant warmer

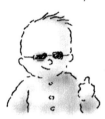

Phototherapy is the treatment of choice for neonatal jaundice.

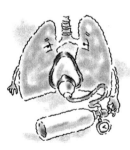

Respiratory distress syndrome occurs most commonly in preterm neonates of diabetic mothers and neonates delivered by cesarean births.

Drug therapy
- Indomethacin (Indocin) to promote closure of the ductus arteriosus (a fetal blood vessel connecting the left pulmonary artery to the descending aorta)

INTERVENTIONS AND RATIONALES
- Assess cardiovascular, respiratory, and neurologic status *for respiratory distress.*
- Monitor vital signs and pulse oximetry readings *to observe for changes.*
- Initiate and maintain ventilatory support status *to maintain air supply.*
- Administer medications, including endotracheal surfactant, as prescribed *to improve respiratory function.*
- Assess hydration status *to assess fluid loss.*
- Maintain I.V. therapy *to maintain fluid levels.*
- Provide adequate nutrition through enteral feedings, if possible, or TPN *to provide adequate nutrition.*
- Maintain thermoregulation *to reduce cold stress.*
- Obtain blood samples, as necessary, *to assess for complications.*

Teaching topics
- Explanation of the disorder and treatment plan
- Promoting maternal-neonatal bonding

Tracheoesophageal fistula

Tracheoesophageal fistula is a congenital anomaly in which the esophagus and trachea don't separate normally. Most commonly, the esophagus ends in a blind pouch, with the trachea communicating by a fistula with the lower esophagus and stomach.

CAUSES
- Abnormal development of the trachea and esophagus during the embryonic period

ASSESSMENT FINDINGS
- Difficulty feeding, such as choking or aspiration; cyanosis during feeding
- Difficulty passing a nasogastric tube
- Excessive mucus secretions
- Maternal polyhydramnios (because fetus can't swallow amniotic fluid)

- Signs of respiratory distress (tachypnea, cyanosis, sternal and substernal retractions)

DIAGNOSTIC TEST RESULTS
- Abdominal X-ray shows the fistula and a gas-free abdomen.
- Bronchoscopy shows a blind pouch.

NURSING DIAGNOSES
- Imbalanced nutrition: Less than body requirements
- Impaired gas exchange
- Risk for aspiration

TREATMENT
- Emergency surgical intervention to prevent pneumonia, dehydration, and fluid and electrolyte imbalances
- Gastrostomy tube placement
- Maintenance of a patent airway

Drug therapy
- Antibiotics (as prophylaxis for aspiration pneumonia)

INTERVENTIONS AND RATIONALES
- Assess cardiovascular, respiratory, and GI status *for complications.*
- Monitor vital signs, fluid intake and output, and transcutaneous blood oxygen tension *to assess fluid replacement needs.*
- Place the neonate in high Fowler's position *to prevent aspiration of gastric contents.*
- Keep a laryngoscope and endotracheal tube at the bedside *in case extreme edema causes obstruction.*
- Provide frequent shallow suctioning for very short periods *to maintain airway patency.*
- Provide the neonate with a pacifier *to meet sucking needs.*
- Provide gastrostomy tube feedings postoperatively *to maintain nutrition.*
- Maintain I.V. fluid therapy *to replace fluid volume.*

Teaching topics
- Explanation of the disorder and treatment plan
- Promoting maternal-neonatal bonding
- Neonatal nutritional needs

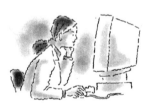

A neonate exhibits difficulty feeding and respiratory distress? That might mean tracheoesophageal fistula.

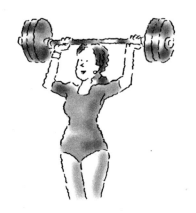

Pump up on practice questions

1. A neonate weighing 1,503 g is born at 32 weeks' gestation. During assessment 12 hours after birth, the nurse notices these signs and symptoms: hyperactivity, persistent shrill cry, frequent yawning and sneezing, and jitteriness. These symptoms indicate:

    1. sepsis.
    2. hepatitis.
    3. drug dependence.
    4. hypoglycemia.

Answer: 3. These classic symptoms of drug dependency usually appear within the first 24 hours after birth. Sepsis is indicated by temperature instability and tachycardia. Hepatitis will manifest itself as jaundice. Hypothermia, muscle twitching, diaphoresis, and respiratory distress may be signs of hypoglycemia.

➥ **NCLEX keys**
Client needs category: Physiological integrity
Client needs subcategory: Physiological adaptation
Cognitive level: Analysis

2. A neonate was delivered 1 hour ago. He's pink with acrocyanosis and exhibits occasional shivering movements of his upper extremities. Which nursing action should take priority?

    1. Obtain vital signs.
    2. Provide warmth with swaddling.
    3. Perform a neurologic assessment.
    4. Evaluate blood glucose.

Answer: 4. A neonate doesn't shiver to increase body temperature; these are jittery movements that indicate hypoglycemia. The blood glucose should be evaluated and addressed with feeding or I.V. glucose. Obtaining vital signs should have been done before this time; if they're due to be repeated, it shouldn't take priority because this will pose a delay in treatment and resolution of low blood glucose. Swaddling may mask the symptoms and doesn't address the underlying issue. Jittery movements don't indicate seizure activity, but unresolved low blood glucose could lead to seizures.

➥ **NCLEX keys**
Client needs category: Safe and effective care environment
Client needs subcategory: Management of care
Cognitive level: Analysis

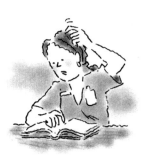

3. A nurse is assessing a 4-hour-old neonate. Which finding should be a cause of concern?

    1. Anterior fontanel is ¾" (1.9 cm) wide, head is molded, and sutures are overriding.
    2. Hands and feet are cyanotic, abdomen is rounded, and the neonate hasn't voided or passed meconium.
    3. Color is dusky, axillary temperature is 97° F (36.1° C), and the neonate is spitting up excessive mucus.
    4. The neonate exhibits irregular abdominal respirations and intermittent tremors in the extremities.

Answer: 3. Skin color is expected to be pink-tinged or ruddy, saliva should be scant, and the normal axillary temperature ranges from

97.7° to 98.6° F (36.5° to 37° C). Overriding sutures and molding, when present, may persist for a few days. Acrocyanosis may be present for 2 to 6 hours. The neonate would be expected to pass meconium and to void within 24 hours. Neonatal tremors are common in a full-term neonate; however, they must be evaluated to differentiate them from seizures.

➥ NCLEX keys

Client needs category: Health promotion and maintenance
Client needs subcategory: None
Cognitive level: Application

4. Which neonate is at greatest risk for developing respiratory distress syndrome?
   1. A neonate with a history of intrauterine growth retardation
   2. A neonate born at less than 35 weeks' gestation
   3. A neonate whose mother experienced prolonged rupture of membranes
   4. A neonate born at 38 weeks' gestation

Answer: 2. Respiratory distress syndrome is predominantly seen in premature neonates; the more premature the neonate, the more severe the disease. Intrauterine growth retardation and prolonged rupture of membranes are unlikely to be associated with the development of respiratory distress syndrome. A 38-week-gestation neonate usually has mature lungs and isn't at risk for respiratory distress syndrome.

➥ NCLEX keys

Client needs category: Physiological integrity
Client needs subcategory: Reduction of risk potential
Cognitive level: Knowledge

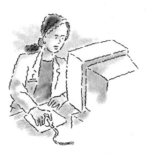

5. A nurse is doing a neurologic assessment on a 1-day-old neonate in the nursery. Which findings indicate possible asphyxia in utero? Select all that apply.
   1. The neonate grasps the nurse's finger when she puts it in the palm of his hand.
   2. The neonate does stepping movements when help upright with the sole of his foot touching a surface.
   3. The neonate's toes don't curl downward when the soles of his feet are stroked.
   4. The neonate doesn't respond when the nurse claps her hands above him.
   5. The neonate turns toward the nurse's finger when she touches his cheek.
   6. The neonate displays weak, ineffective sucking.

Answer: 3, 4, 6. If the neonate's toes don't curl downward when the soles of his feet are stroked and he doesn't respond to a loud sound, it may be evidence that neurologic damage from asphyxia has occurred. A normal neurologic response would be the toes curling downward with stroking and the extension of his arms and legs with a loud noise. Weak, ineffective sucking is another sign of neurologic damage. A neonate should grasp a person's finger when it's placed in the palm of his hand, do stepping movements when help upright with the sole of a foot touching a surface, and turn toward the nurse's finger when she touches his cheek.

➥ NCLEX keys

Client needs category: Health promotion and maintenance
Client needs subcategory: None
Cognitive level: Application

6. A nurse assesses a neonate's respiratory rate at 46 breaths/minute 6 hours after birth. Respirations are shallow, with periods of apnea lasting up to 5 seconds. Which action should the nurse take next?
   1. Attach an apnea monitor.
   2. Continue routine monitoring.
   3. Follow respiratory arrest protocol.
   4. Call the pediatrician immediately to report findings.

Answer: 2. The normal respiratory rate is 30 to 60 breaths/minute. Attaching the apnea monitor, following respiratory arrest protocol, and notifying the pediatrician of findings aren't necessary because the listed findings are normal respiratory patterns in neonates.

➡ *NCLEX keys*

Client needs category: Health promotion and maintenance
Client needs subcategory: None
Cognitive level: Application

7. Which statement is true?
    1. Binge drinking is less detrimental to the fetus than low-level chronic drinking.
    2. The mother's blood alcohol level is greater than that of the fetus.
    3. The fetus can stay inebriated for many days.
    4. Fetal blood alcohol levels drop off quickly.

Answer: 3. The fetal liver isn't mature enough to detoxify the alcohol. Binge drinking is more detrimental to the fetus than chronic low-level drinking for this reason as well. Alcohol goes directly from mother to fetus at the same level of concentration. High fetal blood alcohol levels stay that way for a long time.

➡ *NCLEX keys*

Client needs category: Physiological integrity
Client needs subcategory: Reduction of risk potential
Cognitive level: Analysis

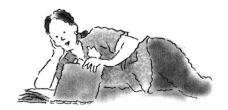

8. The best way to prevent fetal alcohol syndrome (FAS) is for a pregnant woman to:
    1. only drink on social occasions.
    2. stop drinking when she becomes pregnant.
    3. decrease alcohol intake while attempting to become pregnant.
    4. abstain from drinking before becoming pregnant and during the entire pregnancy.

Answer: 4. The best prevention is to abstain from alcohol before and during pregnancy. Social drinking can have adverse effects on an unborn child. Because the fetus can be damaged before the mother realizes that she's pregnant, stopping drinking after the pregnancy becomes known may not prevent FAS. Decreasing alcohol intake may not prevent intrauterine growth retardation.

➡ *NCLEX keys*

Client needs category: Health promotion and maintenance
Client needs subcategory: None
Cognitive level: Analysis

9. A baby girl delivered at 38 weeks' gestation weighs 2,325 g (5 lb, 2 oz) and is having difficulty maintaining body temperature. Which nursing action would best prevent cold stress?
    1. Immediately after birth, dry the neonate and place her under a radiant warmer for 2 hours.
    2. Administer oxygen for the first 30 minutes after birth.
    3. Decrease integumentary stimulation after birth.
    4. Maintain the environmental temperature at a constant level.

Answer: 1. Drying the neonate and placing her in a radiant warmer helps prevent loss of body heat. Administering oxygen and decreasing integumentary circulation would have no effect in preventing cold stress. Maintaining environmental temperature wouldn't prevent loss of heat via conduction, evaporation, or convection.

➡ *NCLEX keys*

Client needs category: Physiological integrity
Client needs subcategory: Physiological adaptation
Cognitive level: Application

10. A nurse is caring for a drug-dependent neonate. Which intervention should the nurse perform?
1. Limit sensory stimulation of the neonate.
2. Cluster activities.
3. Wrap the neonate loosely in blankets.
4. Increase environmental stimuli.

Answer: 1. Limiting sensory stimulation allows for extensive rest periods. The nurse may want to modulate sensory input as tolerated by the neonate. The neonate needs to be swaddled tightly in a flexed position. Increasing environmental stimuli may exacerbate irritability and restlessness.

➡ *NCLEX keys*

Client needs category: Physiological integrity
Client needs subcategory: Physiological adaptation
Cognitive level: Application

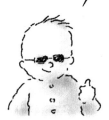

Beautiful. You finished another chapter. Way to goo goo!

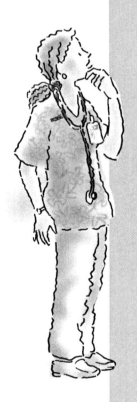

Part III Questions & answers

7   Antepartum care   105

8   Intrapartum care   123

9   Postpartum care   141

10 Neonatal care   159

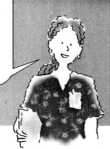

Chapter 7
Antepartum care

1. During an examination, a client who's 32 weeks pregnant becomes dizzy, lightheaded, and pale. While the client is lying supine, which nursing intervention should take <u>priority</u>?
   1. Listen to fetal heart tones.
   2. Take the client's blood pressure.
   3. Ask the client to breathe deeply.
   4. Turn the client on her left side.

Which intervention is of primary importance?

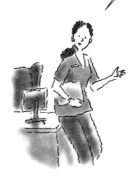

1. 4. As the enlarging uterus increases pressure on the inferior vena cava, it compromises venous return, which can cause dizziness, light-headedness, and pallor when the client is supine. The nurse can relieve these symptoms by turning the client on her left side, which relieves pressure on the vena cava and restores venous return. Although they're valuable assessments, fetal heart tone and maternal blood pressure measurements don't correct the problem. Because deep breathing has no effect on venous return, it can't relieve the client's symptoms.
CN: Safe, effective care environment; CNS: Management of care; CL: Analysis

2. A nurse is assessing a client at 33 weeks' gestation. Leopold's maneuvers indicate that the fetus is in a breech position. Which is the best location for the nurse to auscultate fetal heart tones?
   1. Midway between the symphysis pubis and the umbilicus
   2. Right lower quadrant of the abdomen
   3. Right upper quadrant of the abdomen
   4. Above the level of the umbilicus

2. 4. When the fetus is in the breech position, fetal heart tones are best heard at or above the level of the umbilicus.
CN: Health promotion and maintenance; CNS: None; CL: Application

3. In twin-to-twin transfusion syndrome, the arterial circulation of one twin is in communication with the venous circulation of the other twin. One fetus is considered the "donor" twin and one becomes the "recipient" twin. Assessment of the recipient twin would most likely show which condition?
   1. Anemia
   2. Oligohydramnios
   3. Polycythemia
   4. Small fetus

Careful. Question 3 asks about the recipient twin, not the donor.

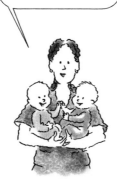

3. 3. The recipient twin in twin-twin transfusion syndrome is transfused by the other twin. The recipient twin then becomes polycythemic and often has heart failure due to circulatory overload. The donor twin becomes anemic. The recipient twin has polyhydramnios, not oligohydramnios. The recipient twin is usually large, whereas the donor twin is often small.
CN: Physiological integrity; CNS: Physiological adaptation; CL: Analysis

---

CN: Client needs category   CNS: Client needs subcategory   CL: Cognitive level

4. A pregnant client who reports painless vaginal bleeding at 28 weeks' gestation is diagnosed with placenta previa. The placental edge reaches the internal os. The nurse would suspect the client has which type of placenta previa?
1. Low-lying placenta previa
2. Marginal placenta previa
3. Partial placenta previa
4. Total placenta previa

5. Expectant management of the client with a placenta implanted in the lower uterine segment includes which procedure or treatment?
1. Stat culture and sensitivity
2. Antenatal steroids after 34 weeks' gestation
3. Ultrasound examination every 2 to 3 weeks
4. Scheduled delivery of the fetus before fetal maturity in a hemodynamically stable mother

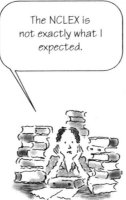

The NCLEX is not exactly what I expected.

6. A client with painless vaginal bleeding at 28 weeks' gestation has just been diagnosed as having placenta previa. Which statement by the client indicates that she understands the nurse's teaching?
1. "I am still able to have sexual intercourse with my husband."
2. "I can continue to go to exercise class three times a week."
3. "I will still be able to fly to Florida for the holidays."
4. "I need to limit my activity and rest."

7. The nurse is teaching a client with placenta previa who has developed placenta accreta. Which statement concerning this condition would be the most correct?
1. The placenta invades the myometrium.
2. The placenta covers the cervical os.
3. The placenta penetrates the myometrium.
4. The placenta attaches to the myometrium.

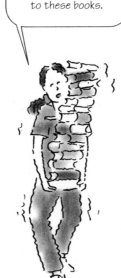

I feel like I'm attached at the hip to these books.

4. 2. A marginal placenta previa is characterized by implantation of the placenta in the margin of the cervical os, not covering the os. A low-lying placenta is implanted in the lower uterine segment but doesn't reach the cervical os. A partial placenta previa is the partial occlusion of the cervical os by the placenta. The internal cervical os is completely covered by the placenta in a total placenta previa.
CN: Physiological integrity; CNS: Physiological adaptation; CL: Analysis

5. 3. Placenta previa occurs when the placenta is implanted in the lower uterine segment. Fetal surveillance through ultrasound examination every 2 to 3 weeks is indicated to evaluate fetal growth, amniotic fluid, and placental location in clients with placenta previa being expectantly managed. A stat culture and sensitivity would be done for severe bleeding or maternal or fetal distress and isn't part of expectant management. Antenatal steroids may be given to clients between 26 and 32 weeks' gestation to enhance fetal lung maturity. In a hemodynamically stable mother, delivery of the fetus should be delayed until fetal lung maturity is attained.
CN: Physiological integrity; CNS: Reduction of risk potential; CL: Analysis

6. 4. The client with placenta previa needs to restrict her activities and may be placed on bed rest. She should avoid sexual intercourse, strenuous activity, and long-distance travel.
CN: Physiological integrity; CNS: Reduction of risk potential; CL: Analysis

7. 4. Placenta accreta is the abnormal attachment of the placenta to the myometrium of the uterus. When the placenta invades the myometrium, it's called placenta increta. When the placenta covers the cervical os, it's called placenta previa. Placenta percreta occurs when the villi of the placenta penetrate the myometrium to the serosa level.
CN: Physiological integrity; CNS: Physiological adaptation; CL: Application

CN: Client needs category   CNS: Client needs subcategory   CL: Cognitive level

8. The nurse is caring for a client suspected of having a hydatidiform mole. Which signs and symptoms would confirm this diagnosis?
1. Heavy, bright red bleeding every 21 days
2. Fetal cardiac motion after 6 weeks' gestation
3. Benign tumors found in the smooth muscle of the uterus
4. "Snowstorm" pattern on ultrasound with no fetus or gestational sac

9. A 21-year-old client has just been diagnosed with having a hydatidiform mole. Which factor is considered a risk factor for developing a hydatidiform mole?
1. Age in 20s or 30s
2. High socioeconomic status
3. Primigravida
4. Prior molar gestation

10. A 21-year-old female client arrives at the emergency department with complaints of cramping, abdominal pain, and mild vaginal bleeding. Pelvic examination shows a left adnexal mass that is tender when palpated. Culdocentesis shows blood in the cul-de-sac. This client probably has which condition?
1. Abruptio placentae
2. Ectopic pregnancy
3. Hydatidiform mole
4. Pelvic inflammatory disease (PID)

11. A client at 34 weeks' gestation arrives at the emergency department with severe abdominal pain, uterine tenderness, and an increased uterine tone. The client denies vaginal bleeding. The external fetal monitor shows fetal distress with severe, variable decelerations. The client most likely has which condition?
1. Abruptio placentae
2. Ectopic pregnancy
3. Molar pregnancy
4. Placenta previa

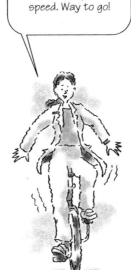

Sometimes it's hard to keep your symptoms straight, isn't it?

Now you're getting up to speed. Way to go!

8. 4. Ultrasound is the technique of choice in diagnosing a hydatidiform mole. The chorionic villi of a molar pregnancy resemble a "snowstorm" pattern on ultrasound. Bleeding with a hydatidiform mole is often dark brown and may occur erratically for weeks or months. There's no cardiac activity because there's no fetus. Benign tumors found in the smooth muscle of the uterus are leiomyomas or fibroids.
CN: Physiological integrity; CNS: Reduction of risk potential; CL: Analysis

9. 4. A previous molar gestation increases a woman's risk for developing a subsequent molar gestation by 4 to 5 times. Adolescents and women ages 40 years and older are at increased risk for molar pregnancies. Multigravidas, especially women with a prior pregnancy loss, and women with lower socioeconomic status are at an increased risk for this problem.
CN: Health promotion and maintenance; CNS: None; CL: Analysis

10. 2. Most ectopic pregnancies don't appear as obvious life-threatening medical emergencies. Ectopic pregnancies must be considered in any sexually active woman of childbearing age who complains of menstrual irregularity, cramping abdominal pain, and mild vaginal bleeding. The client with an ectopic pregnancy who is experiencing blood loss will have blood in the cul-de-sac. PID, abruptio placentae, and hydatidiform moles won't show blood in the cul-de-sac.
CN: Physiological integrity; CNS: Reduction of risk potential; CL: Analysis

11. 1. A client with severe abruptio placentae will often have severe abdominal pain. The uterus will have increased tone with little to no return to resting tone between contractions. The fetus will start to show signs of distress, with decelerations in the heart rate or even fetal death with a large placental separation. An ectopic pregnancy, which usually occurs in the fallopian tubes, would rupture well before 34 weeks. A molar pregnancy generally would be detected before 34 weeks' gestation and no fetal heart sounds would be present. Placenta previa usually involves painless vaginal bleeding without uterine contractions.
CN: Physiological integrity; CNS: Reduction of risk potential; CL: Analysis

12. During a routine visit to the clinic, a client tells the nurse that she thinks she may be pregnant. The physician orders a pregnancy test. Which result would <u>most</u> accurately confirm pregnancy?
1. Increase in human chorionic gonadotropin (HCG)
2. Decrease in HCG
3. Increase in luteinizing hormone (LH)
4. Decrease in LH

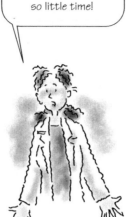

So many hormones to learn; so little time!

12. 1. HCG increases in a woman's blood and urine to fairly large concentrations until the 15th week of pregnancy. The other hormone values aren't indicative of pregnancy.
CN: Health promotion and maintenance; CNS: None; CL: Application

13. A nurse is assessing a pregnant client. Which symptom should the nurse expect to observe?
1. Increased tidal volume
2. Increased expiratory volume
3. Decreased inspiratory capacity
4. Decreased oxygen consumption

13. 1. A pregnant client breathes deeper, which increases the tidal volume of gas moved in and out of the respiratory tract with each breath. The expiratory volume and residual volume decrease as the pregnancy progresses. The inspiratory capacity increases during pregnancy. The increased oxygen consumption in the pregnant client is 15% to 20% greater than in the nonpregnant state.
CN: Health promotion and maintenance; CNS: None; CL: Application

14. Which intervention should the nurse implement in the client scheduled for amniocentesis?
1. Tell the client to drink 1L of water.
2. Have the client void.
3. Instruct the client to fast for 12 hours.
4. Place the client on her left side.

14. 2. Before amniocentesis, the client should void to empty the bladder, reducing the risk of bladder perforation. The client doesn't need to drink fluids before amniocentesis nor does she need to fast. The client should be placed in a supine position for the procedure.
CN: Health promotion and maintenance; CNS: None; CL: Application

15. A nurse is taking an initial history on a pregnant client, who asks about the chances of having dizygotic twins. Which statement by the nurse is correct?
1. "They occur most frequently in Asian women."
2. "There's a decreased risk with increased parity."
3. "There's an increased risk with increased maternal age."
4. "There's no increased risk with the use of fertility drugs."

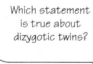

Which statement is true about dizygotic twins?

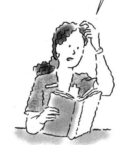

15. 3. Dizygotic twinning is influenced by race (most frequent in Black women and least frequent in Asian women), age (increased risk with increased maternal age), parity (increased risk with increased parity), and fertility drugs (increased risk with the use of fertility drugs, especially ovulation-inducing drugs). The incidence of monozygotic twins isn't affected by race, age, parity, heredity, or fertility medications.
CN: Health promotion and maintenance; CNS: None; CL: Application

CN: Client needs category   CNS: Client needs subcategory   CL: Cognitive level

16. A client in her fifth month of pregnancy is having a routine clinic visit. The nurse should assess the client for which common <u>second</u> trimester condition?
1. Mastitis
2. Metabolic alkalosis
3. Physiologic anemia
4. Respiratory acidosis

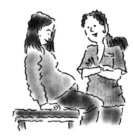

A pregnant client's needs may vary in each trimester.

16. 3. Hemoglobin and hematocrit values decrease during pregnancy as the increase in plasma volume exceeds the increase in red blood cell production. Mastitis is an infection in the breast characterized by a swollen tender breast and flulike symptoms. This condition is most frequently seen in breast-feeding clients. Alterations in acid-base balance during pregnancy result in a state of respiratory alkalosis, compensated by mild metabolic acidosis.
CN: Health promotion and maintenance; CNS: None; CL: Application

17. A 21-year-old client at 6 weeks' gestation is diagnosed with hyperemesis gravidarum. This excessive vomiting during pregnancy will often result in which condition?
1. Bowel perforation
2. Electrolyte imbalance
3. Miscarriage
4. Gestational hypertension

17. 2. Excessive vomiting in clients with hyperemesis gravidarum often causes weight loss and fluid, electrolyte, and acid-base imbalances. Clients with severe hyperemesis may have a low-birth-weight infant, but the disorder generally isn't life-threatening to the fetus. Gestational hypertension and bowel perforation aren't related to hyperemesis. The effects of hyperemesis on the fetus depend on the severity of the disorder.
CN: Physiological integrity; CNS: Reduction of risk potential; CL: Analysis

18. A 29-year-old client has gestational diabetes. The nurse is teaching her about managing her glucose levels. Which therapy would be most appropriate for this client?
1. Diet
2. Long-acting insulin
3. Oral hypoglycemic drugs
4. Glucagon

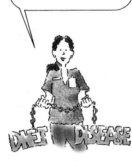

Clients with gestational diabetes need nutritional counseling.

DIET DISEASE

18. 1. Clients with gestational diabetes are usually managed by diet alone to control their glucose intolerance. Long-acting insulin usually isn't needed for blood glucose control in the client with gestational diabetes. Oral hypoglycemic drugs are contraindicated in pregnancy. Glucagon raises blood glucose and is used to treat hypoglycemic reactions.
CN: Health promotion and maintenance; CNS: None; CL: Application

19. Magnesium sulfate is given to pregnant clients with preeclampsia to prevent which condition?
1. Hemorrhage
2. Hypertension
3. Hypomagnesemia
4. Seizures

19. 4. The anticonvulsant mechanism of magnesium is believed to depress seizure foci in the brain and peripheral neuromuscular blockade. Magnesium doesn't help prevent hemorrhage in preeclamptic clients. Anti-hypertensive drugs other than magnesium are preferred for sustained hypertension. Hypomagnesemia isn't a complication of preeclampsia.
CN: Physiological integrity; CNS: Pharmacological and parenteral therapies; CL: Analysis

20. While assessing a client in her 24th week of pregnancy, the nurse learns that the client has been experiencing signs and symptoms of pregnancy-induced hypertension, or preeclampsia. Which sign or symptom helps differentiate preeclampsia from eclampsia?
1. Seizures
2. Headaches
3. Blurred vision
4. Weight gain

21. A pregnant client has a negative contraction stress test (CST). Which statement most accurately describes these test results?
1. Persistent late decelerations in fetal heartbeat occurred, with at least three contractions in a 10-minute window.
2. Accelerations of fetal heartbeat occurred, with at least 15 beats/minute, lasting 15 to 30 seconds in a 20-minute period.
3. Accelerations of fetal heartbeat were absent or didn't increase by 15 beats/minute for 15 to 30 seconds in a 20-minute period.
4. There was good fetal heart rate (FHR) variability and no decelerations from contraction in a 10-minute period in which there were three contractions.

22. A pregnant client with sickle cell anemia is at an increased risk for having a sickle cell crisis during pregnancy. Aggressive management of a sickle cell crisis includes which measure?
1. Antihypertensive agents
2. Diuretic agents
3. I.V. fluids
4. Acetaminophen (Tylenol) for pain

23. A nurse is assessing a pregnant client. Which cardiac condition should the nurse realistically expect in a normal pregnancy?
1. Cardiac tamponade
2. Heart failure
3. Endocarditis
4. Systolic murmur

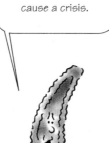

I didn't mean to cause a crisis.

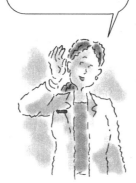

I think I hear the answer to question 23.

20. 1. The primary difference between preeclampsia and eclampsia is the occurrence of seizures, which occur when the client becomes eclamptic. Headaches, blurred vision, weight gain, increased blood pressure, and edema of the hands and feet are all indicative of preeclampsia.
CN: Physiological integrity; CNS: Physiological adaptation; CL: Application

21. 4. A CST measures the fetal response to uterine contractions. A client must have three contractions in a 10-minute period. A negative CST shows good FHR variability with no decelerations from uterine contractions. Persistent late decelerations with contractions is a positive CST. Reactive NSTs have accelerations in the fetal heartbeat of at least 15 beats/minute lasting 15 to 30 seconds in a 20-minute period. No accelerations in the heartbeat of at least 15 beats/minute for 15 to 30 seconds in a 20 minute period indicate a nonreactive nonstress test (NST).
CN: Physiological integrity; CNS: Reduction of risk potential; CL: Analysis

22. 3. A sickle cell crisis during pregnancy is usually managed by exchange transfusion, oxygen, and I.V. fluids. Antihypertensive drugs usually aren't necessary. Diuretics wouldn't be used unless fluid overload resulted. The client usually needs a stronger analgesic than acetaminophen to control the pain of a crisis.
CN: Physiological integrity; CNS: Reduction of risk potential; CL: Analysis

23. 4. Systolic murmurs are heard in up to 90% of pregnant clients, and the murmur disappears soon after the delivery. Cardiac tamponade, which causes effusion of fluid into the pericardial sac, isn't normal during pregnancy. Despite the increases in intravascular volume and workload of the heart associated with pregnancy, heart failure isn't normal in pregnancy. Endocarditis is most often associated with I.V. drug use and isn't a normal finding in pregnancy.
CN: Health promotion and maintenance; CNS: None; CL: Application

24. A 42-year-old pregnant client presents for her first prenatal visit at 16 weeks' gestation. She has severe morning sickness and no fetal heart tones. Her B/P is 150/100. Fundal height is 24 cm. These signs are most likely indicative of which condition?
1. Abruptio placenta
2. Placenta previa
3. Normal pregnancy
4. Hydatidiform mole

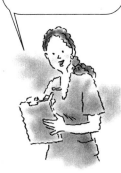

The words *most likely* can help you focus on the correct answer.

25. A client with gestational hypertension is receiving magnesium sulfate to prevent seizure activity. Which magnesium level is therapeutic for clients with preeclampsia?
1. 4 to 7 mEq/L
2. 8 to 10 mEq/L
3. 10 to 12 mEq/L
4. Greater than 15 mEq/L

26. A client is receiving I.V. magnesium sulfate for severe preeclampsia. Which adverse effect is associated with magnesium sulfate?
1. Anemia
2. Decreased urine output
3. Hyperreflexia
4. Increased respiratory rate

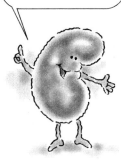

With the right drug, I can get rid of that extra magnesium.

27. The antagonist for magnesium sulfate should be readily available to any client receiving I.V. magnesium. Which drug is the antidote for magnesium toxicity?
1. Calcium gluconate (Kalcinate)
2. Hydralazine
3. Naloxone
4. $Rh_0(D)$ immune globulin (RhoGAM)

24. 4. The incidence of hydatidiform mole, also known as gestational trophoblastic disease, is higher in women who are older than 35 years of age, have low protein intake, or of Asian heritage. Molar pregnancy should be suspected in clients who have bleeding during the first half of pregnancy, hyperemesis, pregnancy-induced hypertension, absent fetal heart tones, and enlarged uterus for the time of pregnancy. The signs and symptoms do not pertain to the other conditions.
CN: Health promotion and maintenance; CNS: None; CL: Application

25. 1. The therapeutic level of magnesium for clients with gestational hypertension is 4 to 7 mEq/L. A serum level of 8 to 10 mEq/L may cause the absence of reflexes in the client. Serum levels of 10 to 12 mEq/L may cause respiratory depression, and a serum level of magnesium greater than 15 mEq/L may result in respiratory paralysis.
CN: Physiological integrity; CNS: Pharmacological and parenteral therapies; CL: Application

26. 2. Decreased urine output may occur in clients receiving I.V. magnesium and should be monitored closely to keep urine output at greater than 30 ml/hour because magnesium is excreted through the kidneys and can easily accumulate to toxic levels. Anemia isn't associated with magnesium therapy. Magnesium infusions may cause depression of deep tendon reflexes or hyporeflexia. The client should be monitored for respiratory depression and paralysis when serum magnesium levels reach approximately 15 mEq/L.
CN: Physiological integrity; CNS: Pharmacological and parenteral therapies; CL: Analysis

27. 1. Calcium gluconate is the antidote for magnesium toxicity. Ten milliliters of 10% calcium gluconate is given I.V. push over 3 to 5 minutes. Hydralazine is given for sustained elevated blood pressures in preeclamptic clients. Naloxone is used to correct narcotic toxicity. $Rh_0(D)$ immune globulin is given to women with Rh-negative blood to prevent antibody formation from Rh-positive conceptions.
CN: Physiological integrity; CNS: Pharmacological and parenteral therapies; CL: Analysis

28. A pregnant client is screened for tuberculosis during her first prenatal visit. An intradermal injection of purified protein derivative (PPD) of the tuberculin bacilli is given. The client is considered to have a positive test for which result?

1. An indurated wheal under 10 mm in diameter appears in 6 to 12 hours.
2. An indurated wheal over 10 mm in diameter appears in 48 to 72 hours.
3. A flat circumcised area under 10 mm in diameter appears in 6 to 12 hours.
4. A flat circumcised area over 10 mm in diameter appears in 48 to 72 hours.

29. A 23-year-old client who is at 27 weeks' gestation arrives at her physician's office with complaints of fever, nausea, vomiting, malaise, unilateral flank pain, and costovertebral angle tenderness. Which diagnosis is most likely?

1. Asymptomatic bacteriuria
2. Bacterial vaginosis
3. Pyelonephritis
4. Urinary tract infection (UTI)

30. Clients with which condition would be appropriate for a trial of labor after a prior cesarean delivery?

1. Complete placenta previa
2. Invasive cervical cancer
3. Premature rupture of membranes
4. Prior classical cesarean delivery

31. A nurse is teaching a client who receives a dose of RhoGAM (human Rh$_0$[D] immune globulin) at 28 weeks' gestation to prevent Rh isoimmunization. Which statement is most accurate about the development of this condition?

1. Rh-positive maternal blood crosses into fetal blood, stimulating fetal antibodies.
2. Rh-positive fetal blood crosses into maternal blood, stimulating maternal antibodies.
3. Rh-negative fetal blood crosses into maternal blood, stimulating maternal antibodies.
4. Rh-negative maternal blood crosses into fetal blood, stimulating fetal antibodies.

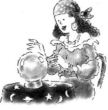

A mysterious wheal will appear within the next few days.

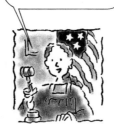

This isn't my kind of trial.

28. 2. A positive PPD result would be an indurated wheal over 10 mm in diameter that appears in 48 to 72 hours. The area must be a raised wheal, not a flat circumcised area, to be considered positive.

CN: Physiological integrity; CNS: Reduction of risk potential; CL: Application

29. 3. The symptoms indicate acute pyelonephritis, a serious condition in a pregnant client. Asymptomatic bacteriuria doesn't cause symptoms. Bacterial vaginosis causes milky white vaginal discharge but no systemic symptoms. UTI symptoms include dysuria, urgency, frequency, and suprapubic tenderness.

CN: Physiological integrity; CNS: Reduction of risk potential; CL: Analysis

30. 3. Clients with premature rupture of membranes are permitted a trial of labor after a previous cesarean delivery. Clients with placenta previa or a prior classical cesarean delivery shouldn't be given a trial of labor due to the risk of uterine rupture or severe bleeding. A client with invasive cervical cancer should be scheduled for a cesarean delivery.

CN: Physiological integrity; CNS: Physiological adaptation; CL: Analysis

31. 2. Rh isoimmunization occurs when Rh-positive fetal blood cells cross into the maternal circulation and stimulate maternal antibody production. In subsequent pregnancies with Rh-positive fetuses, maternal antibodies may cross back into the fetal circulation and destroy the fetal blood cells.

CN: Physiological integrity; CNS: Reduction of risk potential; CL: Application

CN: Client needs category   CNS: Client needs subcategory   CL: Cognitive level

32. Which dose of $Rh_0(D)$ immune globulin (RhoGAM) is appropriate for a pregnant client at 28 weeks' gestation?
1. 50 mcg in a sensitized client
2. 50 mcg in an unsensitized client
3. 300 mcg in a sensitized client
4. 300 mcg in an unsensitized client

33. A client hospitalized for preterm labor tells the nurse she's having occasional contractions. Which nursing intervention would be the <u>most appropriate</u>?
1. Teach the client the possible complications of preterm birth.
2. Tell the client to walk to see if she can get rid of the contractions.
3. Encourage her to empty her bladder and drink plenty of fluids, and give I.V. fluids.
4. Notify anesthesia for immediate epidural placement to relieve the pain associated with contractions.

34. A client's prenatal history shows her to be a 23-year-old gravida 4, para 2. The nurse has correctly interpreted this information when she makes which statement?
1. "The client has been pregnant four times and has had two miscarriages."
2. "The client has been pregnant four times and has had two children born after 20 weeks' gestation."
3. "The client has been pregnant four times and has had two cesarean deliveries."
4. "The client has been pregnant four times and has had two spontaneous abortions."

35. A nurse is planning the care of a pregnant client. Which condition would require more frequent visits?
1. Blood type O positive
2. First pregnancy at age 33 years
3. History of allergy to honey bee pollen
4. History of insulin-dependent diabetes mellitus

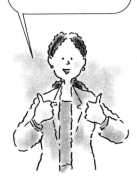

It may be premature. But I think you're doing great!

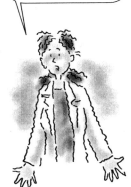

Nobody told me that I'd have to know Latin!

32. 4. An Rh-negative unsensitized woman should be given 300 mcg of RhoGAM at 28 weeks' gestation after an indirect Coombs, test is done to verify that sensitization hasn't occurred. For a first-trimester abortion or ectopic pregnancy, 50 mcg of RhoGAM is given. The administration of RhoGAM to a sensitized client isn't effective.
CN: Physiological integrity; CNS: Pharmacological and parenteral therapies; CL: Analysis

33. 3. An empty bladder and adequate hydration may help decrease or stop labor contractions. Teaching the potential complications is likely to increase the client's anxiety rather than help her relax. Walking may encourage contractions to become stronger. It would be inappropriate to call anesthesia and have an epidural placed because further assessment of contractions is necessary.
CN: Physiological integrity; CNS: Reduction of risk potential; CL: Application

34. 2. *Gravida* refers to the number of times a client has been pregnant; *para* refers to the number of viable children born after 20 weeks' gestation. Therefore, the client who is *gravida 4, para 2* has been pregnant four times and had two live-born children.
CN: Health promotion and maintenance; CNS: None; CL: Analysis

35. 4. A woman with a history of diabetes has an increased risk for perinatal complications, including hypertension, preeclampsia, and neonatal hypoglycemia and, therefore, needs to be more closely monitored. The age of 33 years without other risk factors doesn't increase risk, nor does type O positive blood or environmental allergens.
CN: Safe, effective care environment; CNS: Management of care; CL: Application

36. To detect life-threatening complications as early as possible in a client receiving a tocolytic agent; the nurse should be alert for which finding?
1. Serum blood glucose level of 140 mg/dl
2. Maternal heart rate of 54 beats/minute
3. Bilateral crackles on lung auscultation
4. Weakened carotid pulse

Some complications require prompt action.

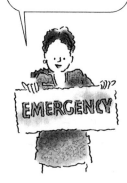

36. 3. Tocolytics are used to stop labor contractions. The most common adverse effect associated with the use of these drugs is pulmonary edema. Therefore, bilateral crackles on lung auscultation, a sign of pulmonary edema, require prompt action. A serum glucose level of 140 mg/dl is elevated and should be reported, however, it isn't life-threatening. Tocolytics may cause tachycardia and increased cardiac output with bounding arterial pulsations.
CN: Physiological integrity; CNS: Pharmacological and parenteral therapies; CL: Analysis

37. What would be the most appropriate medication to administer for a client who has been in early labor (contractions every 10–12 minutes) for 12 hours without progression to help stimulate uterine contractions?
1. Estrogen
2. Fetal cortisol
3. Oxytocin
4. Progesterone

37. 3. Oxytocin is the hormone responsible for stimulating uterine contractions. Pitocin, the synthetic form, may be given to clients to induce or augment uterine contractions. Although estrogen has a role in uterine contractions, it isn't given in a synthetic form to help uterine contractility. Fetal cortisol is believed to slow the production of progesterone by the placenta. Progesterone has a relaxing effect on the uterus.
CN: Physiological integrity; CNS: Pharmacological and parenteral therapies; CL: Application

38. A pregnant client asks the nurse about the pregnancy stage in which maternal and fetal blood are exchanged. Which response by the nurse would be most accurate?
1. Conception
2. 9 weeks' gestation, when the fetal heart is well developed
3. 32 to 34 weeks' gestation (third trimester)
4. Maternal and fetal blood are never exchanged

38. 4. Only nutrients and waste products are transferred across the placenta. Blood exchange never occurs. Complications and some medical procedures can cause an exchange to occur accidentally.
CN: Physiological integrity; CNS: Physiological adaptation; CL: Application

39. Which rationale best explains why a pregnant client should lie on her left side when resting or sleeping in the later stages of pregnancy?
1. To facilitate digestion
2. To facilitate bladder emptying
3. To prevent compression of the vena cava
4. To avoid the development of fetal anomalies

The resting or sleeping position is important in the later stages of pregnancy.

39. 3. The weight of the pregnant uterus is sufficiently heavy to compress the vena cava, which could impair blood flow to the uterus, possibly decreasing oxygen to the fetus. The side-lying position hasn't been shown to prevent fetal anomalies, nor does it facilitate bladder emptying or digestion.
CN: Physiological integrity; CNS: Reduction of risk potential; CL: Analysis

CN: Client needs category   CNS: Client needs subcategory   CL: Cognitive level

40. A pregnant client is concerned about lack of fetal movement. What instructions should the nurse give that might offer reassurance?
   1. Start taking two prenatal vitamins.
   2. Take a warm bath to facilitate fetal movement.
   3. Eat foods that contain a high sugar content to enhance fetal movement.
   4. Lie down once a day and count the number of fetal movements for 15 to 30 minutes.

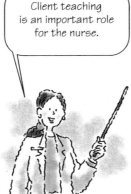

Client teaching is an important role for the nurse.

40. 4. Having the client lie down once during the day will allow her to concentrate on detecting fetal movement, which can be reassuring. Additionally, when the mother is up and actively walking around, it tends to be soothing to the fetus, resulting in sleep promotion. Lying down will make it easier for the client to detect movement. Instructing her to take additional prenatal vitamins isn't recommended as vitamins can be toxic when taken in excess. Taking a warm bath is also likely to be soothing to the fetus. There's also a risk for hyperthermia if the water is too warm or the client is immersed too long. Eating additional sugary foods isn't recommended as some pregnant clients are more susceptible to cavities.
CN: Health promotion and maintenance; CNS: None; CL: Application

41. What would be the most appropriate recommendation to a pregnant client who complains of swelling in her feet and ankles?
   1. Limit fluid intake.
   2. Buy walking shoes.
   3. Sit and elevate the feet.
   4. Start taking a diuretic as needed daily.

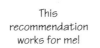

This recommendation works for me!

41. 3. Sitting down and putting up her feet will promote venous return and therefore decrease edema. Limiting fluid intake isn't recommended unless there are additional medical complications such as heart failure. Buying walking shoes won't necessarily decrease edema. Diuretics aren't recommended during pregnancy because it's important to maintain an adequate circulatory volume.
CN: Physiological integrity; CNS: Basic care and comfort; CL: Application

42. Which intervention should a nurse recommend to a client having severe heartburn during her pregnancy?
   1. Eat several small meals daily.
   2. Eat crackers on waking every a.m.
   3. Drink a preparation of salt and vinegar.
   4. Drink orange juice frequently during the day.

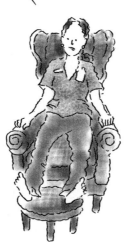

42. 1. Eating small frequent meals will place less pressure on the esophageal sphincter, reducing the likelihood of the regurgitation of stomach contents into the lower esophagus. None of the other suggestions have been shown to decrease heartburn.
CN: Physiological integrity; CNS: Basic care and comfort; CL: Application

43. Which maternal complication is associated with obesity in pregnancy?
   1. Mastitis
   2. Placenta previa
   3. Preeclampsia
   4. Rh isoimmunization

43. 3. The incidence of preeclampsia in obese clients is about seven times more than that in nonobese pregnant clients. Mastitis, placenta previa, and Rh isoimmunization aren't associated with increased incidence in obese pregnant clients.
CN: Physiological integrity; CNS: Reduction of risk potential; CL: Analysis

44. Because uteroplacental circulation is compromised in clients with preeclampsia, a nonstress test (NST) is performed to assess which condition?
1. Anemia
2. Fetal well-being
3. Intrauterine growth retardation (IUGR)
4. Oligohydramnios

45. A client is at 33 weeks' gestation and has had diabetes since she was 21. When checking her fasting blood sugar level, which value would indicate the client's disease was controlled?
1. 45 mg/dl
2. 85 mg/dl
3. 120 mg/dl
4. 136 mg/dl

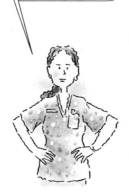

It's important to know the recommended fasting blood sugar level during pregnancy.

46. A client with diabetes, who is in the late third trimester, has a nonstress test twice weekly. The 20-minute test showed three fetal heart rate accelerations that exceeded the baseline by 15 beats/minute and that lasted longer than 15 seconds. The nurse knows these results are consistent with which interpretation of a nonstress test?
1. Reactive test
2. Nonreactive test
3. Positive test
4. Negative test

47. A client is diagnosed with preterm labor at 28 weeks' gestation. Later, she comes to the emergency department saying, "I think I'm in labor." The nurse should expect her physical examination to show which condition?
1. Painful contractions with no cervical dilation
2. Regular uterine contractions with cervical dilation
3. Irregular uterine contraction with no cervical dilation
4. Irregular uterine contractions with cervical effacement

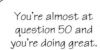

You're almost at question 50 and you're doing great.

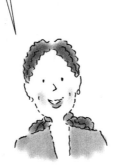

44. 2. An NST is based on the theory that a healthy fetus will have transient fetal heart rate accelerations with fetal movement. A fetus with compromised uteroplacental circulation usually won't have these accelerations, which indicate a nonreactive NST. An NST can't detect anemia in a fetus. Serial ultrasounds will detect IUGR and oligohydramnios in a fetus.
CN: Health promotion and maintenance; CNS: None; CL: Analysis

45. 2. Recommended fasting blood sugar levels in pregnant clients with diabetes are 60 to 90 mg/dl. A fasting blood sugar level of 45 mg/dl is low and may result in symptoms of hypoglycemia. A blood sugar level below 120 mg/dl is recommended for 1-hour postprandial values. A blood sugar level above 136 mg/dl in a pregnant client indicates hyperglycemia.
CN: Health promotion and maintenance; CNS: None; CL: Analysis

46. 1. The nonstress test is the preferred antepartum heart-rate screening test for pregnant clients with diabetes. A reactive nonstress test is two or more fetal heart rate accelerations that exceed the baseline by at least 15 beats/minute and that last longer than 15 seconds within a 20-minute period. A nonreactive nonstress test lacks accelerations in the fetal heart rate with fetal movement. The terms positive and negative aren't used to describe the interpretation of nonstress tests.
CN: Physiological integrity; CNS: Reduction of risk potential; CL: Analysis

47. 2. Regular uterine contractions (every 10 minutes or more) along with cervical dilation change before 36 weeks is considered preterm labor. No cervical change with uterine contractions isn't considered preterm labor.
CN: Health promotion and maintenance; CNS: None; CL: Application

48. A client at 18 weeks' gestation reports fluttering sensations in her abdomen. Which statement made by the client indicates that the nurse's teaching was successful?
1. "This is my baby moving."
2. "I will seek prompt medical attention if this happens again."
3. "This is an early sign of labor."
4. "I will avoid spicy foods."

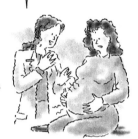

Oh my! I think your baby just moved.

49. A pregnant client is visiting the clinic and complains about the tiny, blanched, slightly raised end arterioles on her face, neck, arms, and chest. The nurse should explain that these are normal during pregnancy and referred to as which finding?
1. Epulis
2. Linea nigra
3. Striae gravidarum
4. Telangiectasias

50. Which nursing intervention for a pregnant adolescent client has the highest priority during the first trimester?
1. Schedule the client for a screening glucose tolerance test.
2. Refer the client to a dietitian for nutritional counseling.
3. Tell the client that she will most likely need a cesarean delivery due to the head size of the fetus.
4. Assess the client for signs and symptoms of placenta previa.

51. A nurse is discussing nutrition with a prima gravida client. The client states that she knows that calcium is important during pregnancy; however, she and her family don't consume many milk or dairy products. What advice should the nurse give?
1. "The prenatal vitamins that are recommended will satisfy all dietary requirements."
2. "You could supplement your diet with 1800 mg of over-the-counter calcium tablets."
3. "You should consume other non-dairy foods that are high in calcium."
4. "After the first trimester, calcium intake isn't significant because all fetal organ structures are formed."

48. 1. Fluttering in the abdomen, also called *quickening,* begins between 16 and 22 weeks' gestation and is caused by fetal movement. It doesn't require medical attention, nor is it a sign of early labor. Eating spicy foods has no effect on quickening.
CN: Health promotion and maintenance; CNS: None; CL: Analysis

49. 4. The dilated arterioles that occur during pregnancy are due to the elevated level of circulating estrogen and are called telangiectasias. An epulis is a red raised nodule on the gums that may develop at the end of the first trimester and continue to grow as the pregnancy progresses. The linea nigra is a pigmented line extending from the symphysis pubis to the top of the fundus during pregnancy. Striae gravidarum, or stretch marks, are slightly depressed streaks that commonly occur over the abdomen, breast, and thighs during the second half of pregnancy.
CN: Health promotion and maintenance; CNS: None; CL: Application

50. 2. Adolescent clients are at risk for delivering low-birth-weight neonates, not macrosomic neonates. Nutritional counseling should be included as part of prenatal care for adolescent clients. The final head size of the fetus is unknown at this time. Adolescents aren't at increased risk for developing gestational diabetes or placenta previa.
CN: Health promotion and maintenance; CNS: None; CL: Analysis

51. 3. Food is considered the ideal source of nutrients. However, milk and dairy aren't the only sources of calcium. While prenatal vitamins are generally recommended, they don't satisfy all requirements. The calcium requirement for pregnancy is 1300 mg/day and over-the-counter supplements aren't always safe and should be specifically recommended by the healthcare practitioner. While it's true that all fetal organs are formed by the end of the first trimester, development continues throughout pregnancy.
CN: Health promotion and maintenance; CNS: None; CL: Application

52. Which drug should a nurse choose to utilize as an antagonist for magnesium sulfate?
1. Oxytocin (Pitocin)
2. Terbutaline
3. Calcium gluconate
4. Naloxone

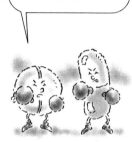

Who are you calling an antagonist?

52. 3. Calcium gluconate should be kept at the bedside while a client is receiving a magnesium infusion. If magnesium toxicity occurs, calcium gluconate is administered as an antidote. Oxytocin is the synthetic form of the naturally occurring pituitary hormone used to initiate or augment uterine contractions. Terbutaline is a beta$_2$-adrenergic agonist that may be used to relax the smooth muscle of the uterus, especially for preterm labor and uterine hyperstimulation. Naloxone is an opiate antagonist administered to reverse the respiratory depression that may follow administration of opiates.
CN: Physiological integrity; CNS: Pharmacological and parenteral therapies; CL: Analysis

53. A nurse receives an order to start an infusion for a client who's hemorrhaging due to a placenta previa. What supplies will be needed?
1. Y tubing, normal saline solution, and a 20G catheter
2. Y tubing, lactated Ringer's solution, and an 18G catheter
3. Y tubing, normal saline solution, and an 18G catheter
4. Y tubing, lactated Ringer's solution, and a 20G catheter

53. 3. Blood transfusions require Y tubing, normal saline solution to mix with the blood product, and an 18G catheter to avoid lysing (breaking) the red blood cells. A 20G catheter lumen isn't large enough for a blood transfusion. Lactated Ringer's solution isn't the I.V. solution of choice with a blood transfusion.
CN: Physiological integrity; CNS: Pharmacological and parenteral therapies; CL: Application

54. Which change should a nurse expect to assess in a client experiencing a normal pregnancy?
1. A 10 beat/minute drop in heart rate
2. A 2 breath/minute increase in respiratory rate
3. A 15 mm Hg increase in systolic blood pressure
4. A 2,000/µl drop in leukocyte count

54. 2. During pregnancy there is a slight increase (2 breaths/minute) in respiratory rate. Heart rate may increase up to 15 beats/minute by the end of pregnancy. Systolic and diastolic pressures may decrease by 5 to 10 mm Hg. The leukocyte count rises in pregnancy and may range from 10,000 to 12,000/µl.
CN: Physiological integrity; CNS: Reduction of risk potential; CL: Application

55. The nurse is teaching a student nurse about the GTPAL system, which documents a client's previous pregnancies. Which statement most accurately describes this system?
  1. Total neonates, Preterm neonates, Anacephalic neonates, and Live births
  2. Total neonates, Problem pregnancies, Abortions, and Live births
  3. Term neonates, Preterm neonates, Anacephalic neonates, and Live births
  4. Term neonates, Preterm neonates, Abortions, and Living children

56. Which glucose tolerance test results in a client at 26 weeks' gestation requires further action?
  1. A glucose level of 120 mg/dl during a 1-hour glucose tolerance test
  2. A 1-hour glucose level of 160 mg/dl during a 3-hour glucose tolerance test
  3. A 2-hour glucose level of 180 mg/dl during a 3-hour glucose tolerance test
  4. A 3-hour glucose level of 130 mg/dl during a 3-hour glucose tolerance test

57. A 32-year-old woman is at 15 weeks' gestation when admitted to the labor unit. According to the GTPAL system, she is a G5 P1212. Which description does this indicate?
  1. Total of 5 pregnancies, 1 full-term pregnancy, 2 problem pregnancies, 1 spontaneous abortion, and 2 live births
  2. Total of 5 children, 1 full-term pregnancy, 2 preterm pregnancies, 1 abortion, 2 live births
  3. Total of 5 pregnancies, 1 full-term pregnancy, 2 preterm pregnancies, 1 abortion, 2 living children
  4. Total of 5 pregnancies, 1 full-term pregnancy, 2 problem pregnancies, 1 abortion, 2 living children

58. Which condition poses the greatest risk to a 32-year-old woman who is 15 weeks' pregnant and has a history of hypertension?
  1. Abruptio placentae
  2. Preterm labor
  3. Spontaneous abortion
  4. Anemia

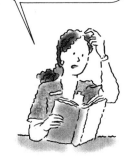

Hmm. Let me think. "G" is for gravida; T is for...

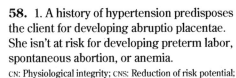

It's important to know the medical history of a pregnant client.

55. 4. In GTPAL, G stands for gravida; T denotes the number of term neonates born after 37 weeks' gestation; P, the number of preterm neonates born before 37 weeks' gestation; A, the number of pregnancies ending with spontaneous or therapeutic abortion; and L, the number of children currently living.
CN: Health promotion and maintenance; CNS: None; CL: Application

56. 2. Gestational diabetes is diagnosed when a 2-hour glucose level is 165 mg/dl or greater during a 3-hour glucose tolerance test. Other abnormal results include a 1-hour glucose tolerance test with a glucose level greater than 140 mg/dl, a 3-hour glucose tolerance test with a 1-hour glucose level of 140 mg/dl or greater, a 3-hour glucose tolerance test with a 2-hour glucose level of 165 mg/dl or greater, or a 3-hour glucose tolerance test with a 3-hour glucose level of 145 mg/dl or greater.
CN: Physiological integrity; CNS: Reduction of risk potential; CL: Application

57. 3. T indicates the number of term neonates born at 37 weeks' gestation or after; P, the number of preterm neonates born before 37 weeks' gestation; A, the number of pregnancies ending with spontaneous or therapeutic abortion; and L, the number of children currently living. In this case, the client has been pregnant five times (including the current pregnancy); has had one pregnancy of at least 37 weeks' gestation, two preterm pregnancies, and one abortion; and has two living children.
CN: Health promotion and maintenance; CNS: None; CL: Application

58. 1. A history of hypertension predisposes the client for developing abruptio placentae. She isn't at risk for developing preterm labor, spontaneous abortion, or anemia.
CN: Physiological integrity; CNS: Reduction of risk potential; CL: Analysis

59. A 32-year-old female client has her first prenatal visit at 15 weeks' gestation. Which finding during this visit is abnormal?
1. Fundal height of 18 cm
2. Blood pressure of 124/72 mm Hg
3. Urine negative for protein
4. Weight of 144 lb (65.3 kg)

Question 59 is asking for an abnormal finding.

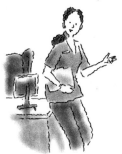

60. A 25-year-old primiparous client arrives for her first prenatal visit at 10 weeks' gestation. She seems nervous and has many questions. Which action should the nurse take first?
1. Assess the client's concerns while taking a comprehensive history.
2. Ask the client to undress to prepare for the physical examination.
3. Reassure the client that all her questions will be answered during the visit.
4. Tell the client there's nothing to worry about; the physician will take care of her.

61. Accompanied by her father, a primiparous 15-year-old client arrives for her first prenatal visit at 30 weeks' gestation. Her father refuses to leave the room, stating that the girl is shy and he will answer the questions for her. Which aspect of this situation should be of most concern to the nurse?
1. The possibility of preterm labor with an adolescent pregnancy
2. Lack of prenatal care until this visit
3. Possible child abuse or domestic violence
4. Difficulties of an overprotective parent in dealing with his daughter

What should the nurse be most concerned about? Let me think.

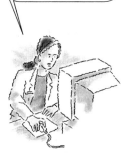

59. 1. Fundal height (in centimeters) should equal the number of weeks' gestation between 18 and 34 weeks; however, it shouldn't be used alone to determine weeks of gestation. This client should have a fundal height of 15 to 16 cm. The blood pressure, urine, and weight findings are within normal limits for the information given.
CN: Physiological integrity; CNS: Reduction of risk potential; CL: Analysis

60. 3. Providing initial reassurance helps set the client's mind at ease. Assessing the client's concerns while taking a history would be appropriate only if the client wrote down her questions in advance. Asking her to disrobe immediately may make the client even more nervous. She should be treated as a partner in her care rather than be told that the physician will take care of everything.
CN: Safe, effective care environment; CNS: Management of care; CL: Application

61. 3. Generally, a father would be somewhat uncomfortable staying in a room while his pregnant daughter is examined. If he insists on staying during the history and physical examination, the nurse should gently but firmly ask him to wait in another room. If the nurse suspects possible child abuse or domestic violence, the father may not want the girl to be alone with the nurse, fearing that she might reveal the abuse or violence. (Typically, a victim of domestic violence says nothing if the perpetrator is in the room with her.) The possibility of preterm labor and lack of prenatal care should be considered— but they aren't the primary concerns in this situation. An overprotective parent can be supported and taught how to let go of a child as time goes by; a social work referral may be warranted.
CN: Psychosocial integrity; CNS: None; CL: Analysis

CN: Client needs category   CNS: Client needs subcategory   CL: Cognitive level

62. Which statement describes the <u>best</u> way for a nurse to determine if a pregnant client is the victim of domestic abuse or violence?
1. Interview the client with her partner in the room.
2. Interview the client with the physician present.
3. Interview the client alone in a nonjudgmental way.
4. Interview the client in a nonjudgmental way, with the partner present.

63. A client with gestational hypertension is experiencing abdominal pain and vaginal bleeding. Which assessment should the nurse perform first?
1. Assess fetal heart tones
2. Assess strength of contractions
3. Assess urinary output
4. Assess serum electrolytes

64. During the second and third trimesters, common pregnancy discomforts may increase in number and severity. Which discomforts would the nurse normally expect to see?
1. Ankle edema, hemorrhoids, nausea and vomiting, and shortness of breath
2. Ankle edema, shortness of breath, leg cramps, and increased vaginal discharge
3. Leg cramps, Braxton Hicks contractions, and nausea and vomiting
4. Leg cramps, ankle edema, and shortness of breath

65. Which statement by a client with mild pre-eclampsia indicates an understanding of discharge instructions?
1. "I will be on my left side."
2. "I should increase my sodium intake."
3. "I will take acetaminophen for a headache."
4. "I will monitor my weight each week."

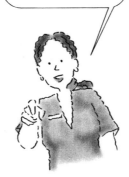

It's up to you to do your best.

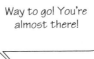

Way to go! You're almost there!

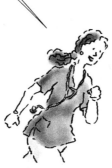

62. 3. To help the client feel protected and develop enough trust in the nurse to share her "secret," the nurse should interview her alone in a nonjudgmental way. If the partner is present, the client is likely to clam up for fear of retaliation the next time they're alone together.
CN: Psychosocial integrity; CNS: None; CL: Application

63. 1. Since the findings suggest that the client is experiencing abruptio placentae, fetal heart tones should immediately be assessed to determine fetal well-being. The other interventions should also be implemented, but after the fetus is assessed.
CN: Physiological integrity; CNS: Reduction of risk potential; CL: Analysis

64. 4. Leg cramps, ankle edema, and shortness of breath are normal during the second and third trimesters. The nurse should teach the client how to relieve minor discomforts and what to report if the discomfort becomes unbearable. Nausea and vomiting should subside by the end of the first trimester; if they don't, the nurse should suspect an undiagnosed problem, such as hyperemesis gravidarum or emotional factors that may be exacerbating the nausea and vomiting. Increased vaginal discharge generally occurs during the first trimester and decreases at the end of this period. A yellow, curdlike, or malodorous discharge suggests an abnormal vaginal infection, which should be reported to the physician.
CN: Health promotion and maintenance; CNS: None; CL: Application

65. 1. The client should lie on her left side to improve uterine and renal blood flow and enhance venous return. Sodium intake should be limited in the client with preeclampsia. A headache should be reported to the health care provider since it can signal a worsening of the eclampsia. Weight should be monitored daily to assess for fluid retention.
CN: Physiological integrity; CNS: Reduction of risk potential; CL: Analysis

66. When teaching an antepartum client about the passage of the fetus through the birth canal during labor, the nurse describes the cardinal mechanisms of labor. Place these events in the proper sequence in which they occur.

| 1. Flexion |
| 2. External rotation |
| 3. Descent |
| 4. Expulsion |
| 5. Internal rotation |
| 6. Extension |

| |
| |
| |
| |
| |
| |

66.

| 3. Descent |
| 1. Flexion |
| 5. Internal rotation |
| 6. Extension |
| 2. External rotation |
| 4. Expulsion |

As the fetus moves through the birth canal, it goes through position changes to ensure that the smallest diameter of fetal head presents to the smallest diameter of the birth canal. Termed the cardinal mechanisms of labor, these position changes occur in the following sequence: descent, flexion, internal rotation, extension, external rotation, and expulsion.

CN: Health promotion and maintenance; CNS: None; CL: Application

67. A nurse is palpating the uterus of a client who is at 20 weeks' gestation to measure fundal height. Identify the area of the abdomen where the nurse should expect to feel the uterine fundus.

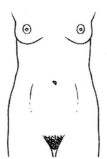

67. At 20 weeks' gestation, fundal height should be at about the umbilicus. Fundal height should be measured from the symphysis pubis to the top of the uterus. Serial measurements assess fetal growth over the course of the pregnancy. Between weeks 18 and 34, the centimeters measured correlate roughly with the week of gestation.

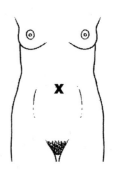

CN: Health promotion and maintenance; CNS: None; CL: Application

CN: Client needs category   CNS: Client needs subcategory   CL: Cognitive level

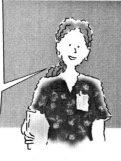

The prepartum and postpartum periods are important to know about. However, the intrapartum period—that's where the action is! This chapter covers the intrapartum period, perhaps the most critical of the three.

Chapter 8
Intrapartum care

1. A client with a term, uncomplicated pregnancy comes into the labor-and-delivery unit in early labor saying that she thinks her water has broken. Which action by a nurse would be <u>most appropriate</u>?
1. Prepare the woman for delivery.
2. Note the color, amount, and odor of the fluid.
3. Immediately contact the physician.
4. Collect a sample of the fluid for microbial analysis.

2. A client who's at 36 weeks' gestation comes into the labor-and-delivery unit with mild contractions. Which complication should a nurse watch for when the client informs her that she has placenta previa?
1. Sudden rupture of membranes
2. Vaginal bleeding
3. Emesis
4. Fever

3. A client's labor doesn't progress. After ruling out cephalopelvic disproportion, the physician orders I.V. administration of 1,000 ml normal saline solution with oxytocin (Pitocin) 10 units to run at 2 milliunits/minute. Two milliunits/minute is equivalent to how many ml/minute?
1. 0.002
2. 0.02
3. 0.2
4. 2

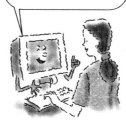

Pay attention to the words *most appropriate*. They're the key to the answer.

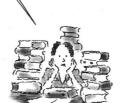

I need a book on math 101.

1. 2. Noting the color, amount, and odor of the fluid, as well as the time of the rupture, will help guide the nurse in her next action. There's no need to call the client's physician immediately or prepare the client for delivery if the fluid is clear and delivery isn't imminent. Rupture of membranes isn't unusual in the early stages of labor. Fluid collection for microbial analysis isn't routine if there's no concern for infection (maternal fever).
CN: Physiological integrity; CNS: Reduction of risk potential; CL: Application

2. 2. Contractions may disrupt the microvascular network in the placenta of a client with placenta previa and result in bleeding. If the separation of the placenta occurs at the margin of the placenta, the blood will escape vaginally. Sudden rupture of the membranes isn't related to placenta previa. Fever would indicate an infectious process, and emesis isn't related to placenta previa.
CN: Physiological integrity; CNS: Reduction of risk potential; CL: Application

3. 3. The answer is found by setting up a ratio and following through with the calculations, shown below. Each unit of oxytocin contains 1,000 milliunits. Therefore, 1,000 ml of I.V. fluid contains 10,000 milliunits (10 units) of Pitocin. All other options are incorrect.

$$\frac{10,000}{1,000} = \frac{2}{X}$$
$$10,000X = 2,000$$
$$X = \frac{2,000}{10,000}$$
$$X = 0.2 \text{ ml}$$

CN: Physiological integrity; CNS: Pharmacological and parenteral therapies; CL: Analysis

CN: Client needs category   CNS: Client needs subcategory   CL: Cognitive level

4. A client in labor has been receiving oxytocin (Pitocin) to aid her progress. The nurse caring for her notes that contractions are lasting 100 seconds. Which action should the nurse take first?
1. Stop the oxytocin infusion.
2. Notify the physician.
3. Monitor fetal heart tones as usual.
4. Turn the client on her left side.

Don't underestimate the importance of the word first.

5. A client at term arrives in the labor unit experiencing contractions every 4 minutes. After a brief assessment, she's admitted and an electriconic fetal monitor is applied. Which observation should alert the nurse to an increased potential for fetal distress?
1. Total weight gain of 30 lb (13.6 kg)
2. Maternal age of 32 years
3. Blood pressure of 146/90 mm Hg
4. Treatment for syphilis at 15 weeks' gestation

6. To detect fetal distress during labor, a nurse should be alert for which finding?
1. Fetal scalp pH of 7.14
2. Fetal heart rate of 144 beats/minute
3. Acceleration of fetal heart rate with contractions
4. Presence of long-term variability

7. During the labor of a client with a breech presentation, the amniotic membranes rupture. Meconium is present in the amniotic fluid. Which statement by a nurse is most appropriate?
1. "This often happens during a prolonged delivery."
2. "This indicates a blood incompatibility between the fetus and mother."
3. "This is a sign of fetal distress."
4. "This is normal in a breech delivery."

4. 1. Oxytocin stimulates contractions and should be stopped. A contraction that continues for more than 90 seconds signals tetany and could lead to decreased placental perfusion and, possibly, uterine rupture. The nurse should monitor the fetal heart tones and notify the physician, but only after stopping the oxytocin. The client should be turned on her left side to increase blood flow to the fetus, which can be decreased with tetany. This decreased blood flow can potentially compromise the fetus.
CN: Physiological integrity; CNS: Reduction of risk potential; CL: Application

5. 3. A blood pressure of 146/90 mm Hg may indicate gestational hypertension. Over time, gestational hypertension reduces blood flow to the placenta and can cause intrauterine growth restriction and other problems that make the fetus less able to tolerate the stress of labor. A weight gain of 30 lb is within expected parameters for a healthy pregnancy. A woman over age 30 doesn't have a greater risk of complications if her general condition is healthy before pregnancy. Syphilis that has been treated doesn't pose an additional risk.
CN: Physiological integrity; CNS: Reduction of risk potential; CL: Application

6. 1. A scalp pH below 7.25 indicates acidosis and fetal hypoxia. A fetal heart rate of 144 beats/minute, acceleration of the fetal heart rate with contractions, and long-term variability are normal responses of a healthy fetus to labor.
CN: Physiological integrity; CNS: Reduction of risk potential; CL: Application

7. 4. Meconium in a breech presentation may be caused by compression of the fetus's intestinal tract during descent. Meconium in the amniotic fluid is a sign of fetal distress in a cephalic presentation and isn't a normal finding, even during a prolonged delivery. Yellow-stained amniotic fluid is a sign of a possible blood incompatibility between fetus and mother and is due to bilirubin from the breakdown of red blood cells.
CN: Physiological integrity; CNS: Reduction of risk potential; CL: Analysis

8. A client at 42 weeks' gestation is 3 cm dilated, 30% effaced, with membranes intact and the fetus at +2 station. Fetal heart rate (FHR) is 140 beats/minute. After 2 hours, the nurse notes on the external fetal monitor that, for the past 10 minutes, the FHR ranged from 160 to 190 beats/minute. The client states that her baby has been extremely active. Uterine contractions are strong, occurring every 3 to 4 minutes and lasting 40 to 60 seconds. Which finding would indicate fetal hypoxia?
1. Abnormally long uterine contractions
2. Abnormally strong uterine intensity
3. Excessively frequent contractions, with rapid fetal movement
4. Excessive fetal activity and fetal tachycardia

9. A client at 33 weeks' gestation and leaking amniotic fluid is placed on an external fetal monitor. The monitor indicates uterine irritability, and contractions are occurring every 4 to 6 minutes. The physician orders terbutaline. Which teaching statement is appropriate for this client?
1. "This medicine will make you breathe better."
2. "You may feel a fluttering or tight sensation in your chest."
3. "This will dry your mouth and make you feel thirsty."
4. "You'll need to replace the potassium lost by this drug."

10. A 17-year-old primigravida with severe hypertension of pregnancy has been receiving magnesium sulfate I.V. for 3 hours. The latest assessment reveals deep tendon reflexes (DTR) of +1, blood pressure of 150/100 mm Hg, a pulse of 92 beats/minute, a respiratory rate of 10 breaths/minute, and urine output of 20 ml/hour. Which action would be most appropriate?
1. Continue monitoring per standards of care.
2. Stop the magnesium sulfate infusion.
3. Increase the infusion rate by 5 gtt/ minute.
4. Decrease the infusion rate by 5 gtt/ minute.

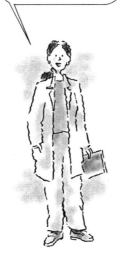

Remember that every piece of information provided may not be necessary to answer the question.

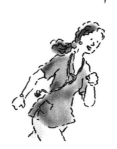

Sometimes you have to think fast on your feet.

8. 4. Fetal tachycardia and excessive fetal activity are the first signs of fetal hypoxia. The duration of uterine contractions is within normal limits. Uterine intensity can be mild to strong and still be within normal limits. The frequency of contractions is within the normal limits for the active phase of labor.
CN: Physiological integrity; CNS: Reduction of risk potential; CL: Analysis

9. 2. A fluttering or tight sensation in the chest is a common adverse reaction to terbutaline. Terbutaline relieves bronchospasm, but the client is receiving it to reduce uterine motility. Mouth dryness and thirst occur with the inhaled form of terbutaline but are unlikely with the subcutaneous form. Hypokalemia is a potential adverse reaction following large doses of terbutaline but not at doses of 0.25 mg.
CN: Health promotion and maintenance; CNS: None; CL: Application

10. 2. Magnesium sulfate should be withheld if the client's respiratory rate or urine output falls or if reflexes are diminished or absent, all of which are true for this client. The client also shows other signs of impending toxicity, such as flushing and feeling warm. Inaction won't resolve the client's suppressed DTRs and low respiratory rate and urine output. The client is already showing central nervous system depression because of excessive magnesium sulfate, so increasing the infusion rate is inappropriate. Impending toxicity indicates that the infusion should be stopped rather than just slowed down.
CN: Physiological integrity; CNS: Pharmacological and parenteral therapies; CL: Application

11. During a vaginal examination of a client in labor, the nurse palpates the fetus's larger, diamond-shaped fontanelle toward the anterior portion of the client's pelvis. Which statement best describes this situation?
1. The client can expect a brief and intense labor with potential for lacerations.
2. The client is at risk for uterine rupture and needs constant monitoring.
3. The client may need interventions to ease back pain and change the fetal position.
4. The fetus will be delivered using forceps or a vacuum extractor.

12. The cervix of a 26-year-old primigravida in labor is 5 cm dilated and 75% effaced, and the fetus is at 0 station. The physician prescribes an epidural regional block. Into which position should the nurse place the client when the epidural is administered?
1. Lithotomy
2. Supine
3. Prone
4. Lateral

13. A nurse administers oxytocin (Pitocin) to a client to induce labor. Which finding should cause the nurse to stop the infusion and notify the physician?
1. Contractions longer than 70 seconds, occurring every 2 minutes or less
2. Dry mucous membranes and decreased skin turgor
3. Fetal heart rate of 160 beats/minute
4. Maternal heart rate of 56 beats/minute

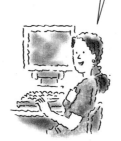

Be careful of the words will be in option 4. They indicate an absolute, a near rarity in health care.

11. 3. The fetal position is occiput posterior, a position that commonly produces intense back pain during labor. Most of the time, the fetus rotates during labor to occiput anterior position. Positioning the client on her side can facilitate this rotation. An occiput posterior position would most likely result in prolonged labor. Occiput posterior alone doesn't create a risk of uterine rupture. The fetus would be delivered with forceps or vacuum extractor only if its presenting part doesn't rotate and descend spontaneously.

CN: Health promotion and maintenance; CNS: None; CL: Analysis

12. 4. The client should be placed on her left side or sitting upright, with her shoulders parallel and legs slightly flexed. Her back shouldn't be flexed because this position increases the possibility that the dura may be punctured and the anesthetic will accidentally be given as spinal, not epidural, anesthesia. None of the other positions allows proper access to the epidural space.

CN: Physiological integrity; CNS: Reduction of risk potential; CL: Application

13. 1. Oxytocin, given to induce labor, may cause uterine tetany, which increases the risk of uterine rupture. Therefore, the infusion should be stopped and the physician notified if contractions last greater than 70 seconds and occur every 2 minutes or less. Oxytocin has an antidiuretic effect and can cause fluid overload, not dehydration indicated by dry mucous membranes and decreased skin turgor. A normal fetal heart rate is 120 to 160 beats/minute. Oxytocin may cause maternal tachycardia, not bradycardia.

CN: Physiological integrity; CNS: Pharmacologic parenteral therapies; CL: Application

CN: Client needs category   CNS: Client needs subcategory   CL: Cognitive level

14. Which fetal position is <u>most favorable</u> for birth?
   1. Vertex presentation
   2. Transverse lie
   3. Frank breech presentation
   4. Posterior position of the fetal head

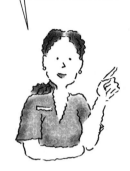

Question 14 is asking for the optimal birthing position.

14. 1. Vertex presentation (flexion of the fetal head) is the optimal presentation for passage through the birth canal. Transverse lie is an unacceptable fetal position for vaginal birth and requires a cesarean birth delivery. Frank breech presentation, in which the buttocks present first, is a high-risk situation and cesarean birth is recommended. Posterior positioning of the fetal head can make it difficult for the fetal head to pass under the maternal symphysis pubis bone.
CN: Physiological integrity; CNS: Reduction of risk potential; CL: Analysis

15. A nurse is preparing a client in the labor-and-delivery unit and is teaching her about the stages of labor. The client demonstrates an understanding of these stages when she states that birth occurs during which stage?
   1. First stage of labor
   2. Second stage of labor
   3. Third stage of labor
   4. Fourth stage of labor

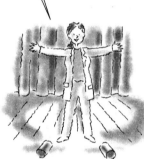

Take the stage please!

15. 2. The second stage of labor begins with complete dilation (10 cm) and ends with the expulsion of the fetus. The first stage of labor is the stage of dilation, which is divided into three distinct phases: latent, active, and transition. The third stage of labor begins with the birth of the infant and ends with the expulsion of the placenta. The fourth stage of labor is the first 4 hours after placental expulsion, in which the client's body begins the recovery process.
CN: Health promotion and maintenance; CNS: None; CL: Application

16. Which laboratory value would be critical for a client admitted to the labor-and-delivery unit?
   1. Blood type
   2. Calcium
   3. Iron
   4. Oxygen saturation

16. 1. Blood type is a critical value to have because the risk of blood loss is always a potential complication during the labor-and-delivery process. Approximately 40% of a woman's cardiac output is delivered to the uterus, therefore, blood loss can occur quite rapidly in the event of uncontrolled bleeding. Calcium and iron aren't critical values and oxygen saturation isn't a laboratory value.
CN: Physiological integrity; CNS: Reduction of risk potential; CL: Analysis

17. Which fetal heart rate would be expected in the fetus of a laboring woman who is full-term?
   1. 80 to 100 beats/minute
   2. 100 to 120 beats/minute
   3. 120 to 160 beats/minute
   4. 160 to 180 beats/minute

17. 3. A rate of 120 to 160 beats/minute in the fetal heart is appropriate for filling the heart with blood and pumping it out to the system. Faster or slower rates don't accomplish perfusion adequately and could indicate fetal compromise.
CN: Health promotion and maintenance; CNS: None; CL: Knowledge

18. A nurse has connected a laboring client to an external electronic fetal monitor. What data can the nurse expect to obtain from the monitor?

1. Gender of the fetus
2. Fetal position
3. Labor progress
4. Oxygenation

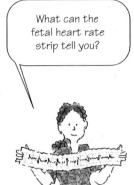

What can the fetal heart rate strip tell you?

19. Which nursing action is required before a client in labor receives an epidural?

1. Give a fluid bolus of 500 ml.
2. Check for maternal pupil dilation.
3. Assess maternal reflexes.
4. Assess maternal gait.

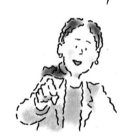

It's important to know the adverse effects of a procedure, and how to offset them.

20. Which complication is possible with an episiotomy?

1. Blood loss
2. Uterine disfigurement
3. Prolonged dyspareunia
4. Hormonal fluctuation postpartum

21. A client in early labor states that she has a thick, yellow discharge from both of her breasts. Which action by the nurse would be most appropriate?

1. Tell her that her milk is starting to come in because she's in labor.
2. Complete a thorough breast examination, and document the results in the chart.
3. Perform a culture on the discharge, and inform the client that she might have mastitis.
4. Inform the client that the discharge is colostrum, normally present after the 4th month of pregnancy.

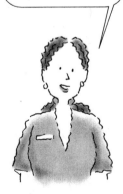

Teaching is an important part of a nurse's role.

18. 4. Oxygenation of the fetus may be indirectly assessed through fetal monitoring by closely examining the fetal heart rate strip. Accelerations in the fetal heart rate strip indicate good oxygenation, while decelerations in the fetal heart rate sometimes indicate poor fetal oxygenation. The fetal heart rate strip can't determine the gender of the fetus or assess fetal position. Labor progress can be directly assessed only through cervical examination.
CN: Physiological integrity; CNS: Reduction of risk potential; CL: Application

19. 1. One of the major adverse effects of epidural administration is hypotension. Therefore, a 500-ml fluid bolus is usually administered to help prevent hypotension in the client who wishes to receive an epidural for pain relief. Assessments of maternal reflexes, pupil response, and gait aren't necessary.
CN: Physiological integrity; CNS: Reduction of risk potential; CL: Analysis

20. 3. Prolonged dyspareunia (painful intercourse) may result when complications such as infection interfere with wound healing. Minimal blood loss occurs when an episiotomy is performed. The uterus isn't affected by episiotomy because it's the perineum that is cut to accommodate the fetus. Hormonal fluctuations that occur during the postpartum period aren't the result of an episiotomy.
CN: Physiological integrity; CNS: Reduction of risk potential; CL: Analysis

21. 4. After the 4th month, colostrum may be expressed. The breasts normally produce colostrum for the first few days after delivery. Milk production begins 1 to 3 days postpartum. A clinical breast examination isn't usually indicated in the intrapartum setting. Although a culture may be indicated, it requires advanced assessment as well as a medical order.
CN: Health promotion and maintenance; CNS: None; CL: Application

CN: Client needs category   CNS: Client needs subcategory   CL: Cognitive level

22. While performing an admission nursing assessment of a client in early labor, the nurse observes a brown, raised lesion resembling a mole, 2″ (5 cm) below the left breast. Which observation by the nurse would be most appropriate?
1. "That looks like a mole and is clinically insignificant."
2. "That looks like seborrhea keratosis and is a precancerous lesion."
3. "That's a supernumerary nipple, a common finding."
4. "That's a skin tag and is clinically insignificant."

23. A client in early labor is concerned about the pinkish "stretch marks" on her abdomen. Which statement by the client indicates that the nurse's teaching has been effective?
1. "My stretch marks will completely fade away within 6 weeks."
2. "My stretch marks will fade but not disappear after delivery."
3. "An emollient cream will help fade my stretch marks."
4. "A regular exercise program will help my stretch marks go away."

24. Which position increases cardiac output and stroke volume of a client in labor?
1. Supine
2. Sitting
3. Side-lying
4. Semi-Fowler's

25. A nurse is caring for a full-term pregnant client in active labor. The electronic fetal monitor reveals a fetal heart rate of less than 70 beats/minute. This finding is considered:
1. Severe fetal bradycardia
2. Normal fetal heart rate
3. Fetal tachycardia
4. Moderate fetal bradycardia

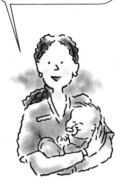

Stretch marks are yet another reminder of the joy of giving birth!

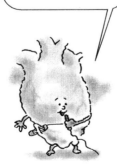

Things are sure getting slow around here.

22. 3. Supernumerary nipples are common in men and women and are usually located 2″ to 2½″ (5 to 6 cm) below the breast near the midline. A supernumerary nipple resembles a mole, although closer inspection will reveal a small nipple and areola and is clinically insignificant. A mole (nevus) may be macular or papular, tan to brown in color, and usually has smooth borders. Keratosis lesions are raised, thickened areas of pigmentation that look scaly and warty. They don't become cancerous. Skin tags (acrochordons) are overgrowths of normal skin that form a stalk and are polyplike.
CN: Health promotion and maintenance; CNS: None; CL: Analysis

23. 2. Striae are wavy, depressed streaks that may occur over the abdomen, breasts, or thighs as pregnancy progresses. They fade with time to a silvery color but won't disappear. Creams may soften the skin but won't remove the striae. Regular exercise won't affect the stretch marks.
CN: Health promotion and maintenance; CNS: None; CL: Application

24. 3. In the side-lying position, cardiac output increases, stroke volume increases, and the pulse rate decreases. In the supine position, the blood pressure can drop severely, due to the pressure of the fetus and enlarged uterus on the vena cava, resulting in supine hypotensive or vena caval syndrome. Neither the sitting nor semi-Fowler's position increases cardiac output or stroke volume.
CN: Health promotion and maintenance; CNS: None; CL: Application

25. 1. A fetal heart rate (FHR) below 70 beats/minute is considered severe fetal bradycardia and is associated with rapidly occurring fetal acidosis. FHR from 70 to 100 beats/minute is considered moderate fetal bradycardia. Normal FHR for a full-term fetus is 120 to 160 beats/minute. Fetal tachycardia is an FHR above 160 beats/minute.
CN: Health promotion and maintenance; CNS: None; CL: Application

26. A nurse is performing Leopold's maneuvers on a client in the early stages of labor. Which finding should alert the nurse to a potential problem?
1. Palpation of the upper fundus reveals a firm, round shape.
2. Palpation of the upper fundus reveals a soft, less-defined shape.
3. Palpation of the side of the fundus reveals a smooth, firm shape.
4. Palpation of the lower fundus reveals a firm, round shape.

27. A client who's at 35 weeks' gestation arrives at a labor-and-delivery unit leaking clear fluid from her vagina. Which intervention would be <u>most appropriate</u>?
1. Perform a cervical examination.
2. Obtain a catheterized urine specimen.
3. Encourage the client to ambulate.
4. Obtain a sterile speculum sample of the fluid.

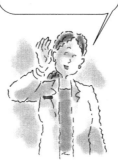

Ah, the sweet sound of most appropriate.

28. A client at 28 weeks' gestation tells the nurse she's having abdominal contractions that started occurring irregularly and have remained irregular. Which statement should the nurse tell the client?
1. "These contractions will disappear when you walk."
2. "These contractions will increase in frequency and intensity."
3. "These contractions will become regular."
4. "These contractions will move to the lower back."

29. While in the first stages of labor, a client with active genital herpes is admitted to the labor-and-delivery area. Which type of birth should the nurse anticipate for this client?
1. Mid-forceps
2. Low forceps
3. Induction
4. Cesarean

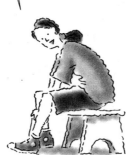

Walking is a great way to relieve stress, and other things!

26. 1. Palpation of the upper fundus reveals a firm, round head in a breech presentation and a soft less-defined shape in a cephalic delivery. The firm, smooth back of the fetus is palpated on the side of the fundus and may be palpated with cephalic and breech presentations. In a cephalic presentation, palpation of the lower fundus reveals a firm, round head.
CN: Health promotion and maintenance; CNS: None; CL: Application

27. 4. A sterile speculum examination is performed to identify ruptured membranes. Confirmation is done with nitrazine paper and a positive ferning test. With premature rupture of membranes in a client under 37 weeks' gestation, cervical examinations are contraindicated to reduce the incidence of infection. Clean catch urine specimens, not catheterized specimens, would be appropriate to rule out infection. The client should ambulate only after a thorough nursing assessment and examination to determine the safety of walking for the client and fetus.
CN: Physiological integrity; CNS: Reduction of risk potential; CL: Application

28. 1. Braxton Hicks contractions begin and remain irregular. They're felt in the abdomen and remain confined to the abdomen and groin. They commonly disappear with ambulation. True contractions begin irregularly but become regular and predictable increasing in frequency and intensity, causing cervical effacement and dilation. True contractions are felt initially in the lower back and radiate to the abdomen in a wavelike motion.
CN: Physiological integrity; CNS: Physiological adaptation; CL: Analysis

29. 4. For a client with active genital herpes, cesarean delivery helps avoid infection transmission to the neonate, which could occur during a vaginal birth. Mid-forceps and low forceps are types of vaginal births that could transmit the herpes infection to the neonate. Induction is used only during vaginal birth; therefore, it's inappropriate for this client.
CN: Physiological integrity; CNS: Reduction of risk potential; CL: Application

CN: Client needs category   CNS: Client needs subcategory   CL: Cognitive level

30. A nurse is monitoring a client in labor and notes on the external fetal monitor that the fetal heart rate (FHR) drops with each contraction. Which action should the nurse take?
1. Turn the client to the left side.
2. Continue to observe FHR.
3. Administer oxygen by face mask.
4. Place the client in Trendelenburg position.

31. The nurse is teaching the stages of labor to a 26-year-old pregnant client. The client would demonstrate that teaching has been effective when she states that crowning occurs during which stage of labor?
1. First
2. Second
3. Third
4. Fourth

32. A nurse suspects that the laboring client may have been physically abused by her male partner. Which intervention by the nurse would be <u>most appropriate</u>?
1. Confront the male partner.
2. Question the woman in front of her partner.
3. Contact hospital security.
4. Collaborate with the physician to make a referral to social services.

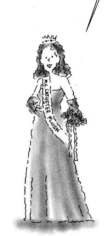

Would you like to know when my crowning took place?

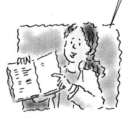

Did you notice the words *most appropriate* in question 32? Another hint!

30. 2. Decelerations in FHR, called *early decelerations,* occur with the onset of uterine contractions. They're caused by head compression during the contraction and aren't a sign of fetal distress. Therefore, no action is necessary and the nurse should continue to monitor the FHR.
CN: Physiological integrity; CNS: Reduction of risk potential; CL: Application

31. 2. The second stage of labor begins at full cervical dilation (10 cm) and ends when the infant is born. Crowning is present during this stage as the fetal head, pushed against the perineum, causes the vaginal introitus to open, allowing the fetal scalp to be visible. The first stage begins with true labor contractions and ends with complete cervical dilation. The third stage is from the time the infant is born until the delivery of the placenta. The fourth stage is the first 1 to 4 hours following delivery of the placenta.
CN: Health promotion and maintenance; CNS: None; CL: Application

32. 4. Collaborating with the physician to make a referral to social services will aid the client by creating a plan and providing support. Additionally, by law, the nurse or nursing supervisor must report the suspected abuse to the police and follow up with a written report. Although confrontation can be used therapeutically, this action will most likely provoke anger in the suspected abuser. Questioning the woman in front of her partner doesn't allow her the privacy required to address this issue and may place her in greater danger. If the woman isn't in imminent danger, there's no need to call hospital security.
CN: Physiological integrity; CNS: Reduction of risk potential; CL: Analysis

33. During a vaginal examination of a client in labor, it is determined that the biparietal diameter of the fetal head has reached the level of the ischial spines. The <u>most accurate</u> documentation of this fetal station would be:
1. −1.
2. 0.
3. +1.
4. +2.

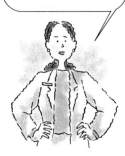

The words most accurate help clarify the correct answer.

33. 2. When the largest diameter of the presenting part (typically the biparietal diameter of the fetal head) is level with the ischial spines, the fetus is at station 0. A station of −1 indicates that the fetal head is 1 cm above the ischial spines. At +1, it's 1 cm below the ischial spines. At +2, it's 2 cm below the ischial spines.

CN: Health promotion and maintenance; CNS: None; CL: Application

34. A nurse has just admitted a client in the labor-and-delivery unit who has been diagnosed by her physician as having diabetes mellitus. Which measure would be most appropriate for this situation?
1. Ask the client about her most recent blood glucose levels.
2. Prepare oral hypoglycemic medications for administration during labor.
3. Notify the neonatal intensive care unit that you've admitted a client with diabetes.
4. Prepare the client for cesarean delivery.

34. 1. As part of the history, asking about the client's most recent blood glucose levels will indicate how well her diabetes has been controlled. Oral hypoglycemic drugs are never used during pregnancy because they cross the placental barrier, stimulate fetal insulin production, and are potentially teratogenic. Plans to admit the infant to the neonatal intensive care unit are premature. Cesarean delivery is no longer the preferred delivery for clients with diabetes. Vaginal birth is preferred and presents a lower risk to the mother and fetus.

CN: Physiological integrity; CNS: Reduction of risk potential; CL: Application

35. A client is admitted to the labor-and-delivery unit with a known anencephalic fetus. Which measure would be appropriate for the nurse to perform?
1. Assess fetal heart tones.
2. Reassure the client that she'll get pregnant again soon.
3. Avoid talking about the baby.
4. Provide privacy.

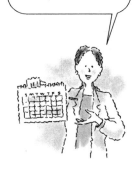

The estimated date of delivery can be determined with the proper information.

35. 4. Providing privacy is an appropriate therapeutic intervention for the client and family to grieve their loss. Fetal heart tones are rarely assessed in a client with an anencephalic fetus; most fetuses won't survive due to lack of cerebral function. Reassuring the client that she will get pregnant again dismisses how she is feeling about her current loss and also provides false reassurance. The nurse should take the lead from the client and family as some people want to talk about their loss and others don't.

CN: Psychosocial integrity; CNS: None; CL: Application

36. A 30-year-old multiparous client admitted to the labor-and-delivery unit hasn't received prenatal care for this pregnancy. Which data is most relevant to the nursing assessment?
1. Date of last menstrual period (LMP)
2. Family history of sexually transmitted diseases (STDs)
3. Name of insurance provider
4. Number of siblings

36. 1. The date of the LMP is essential to estimate the date of delivery. The nursing history would also include subjective information, such as personal (but not necessarily family) history of STDs, gravidity, and parity. Although beneficial to the hospital for financial reimbursement, the insurance provider has no bearing on the nursing history. Likewise, the number of siblings isn't pertinent to the assessment.

CN: Health promotion and maintenance; CNS: None; CL: Analysis

37. Which symptom, when observed in laboring clients with hypertension of pregnancy, would <u>most likely</u> indicate a worsening condition?
1. Decreasing blood pressure
2. Increasing oliguria
3. Decreasing edema
4. Trace levels of protein in the urine

38. While performing a cervical examination, a nurse's fingertips feel pulsating tissue. What would be the most appropriate nursing intervention?
1. Leave the client and call the physician.
2. Put the client in a semi-Fowler's position.
3. Ask the client to push with the next contraction.
4. Leave the fingers in place and press the nurse call light.

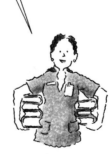

Question 39 is asking you to prioritize!

39. A client is admitted to the labor-and-delivery unit in labor, with blood flowing down her legs. Which nursing intervention would be <u>most appropriate</u>?
1. Place an indwelling catheter.
2. Monitor fetal heart tones.
3. Perform a cervical examination.
4. Prepare the client for cesarean delivery.

37. 2. Renal plasma flow and glomerular filtration are decreased in gestational hypertension, so increasing oliguria indicates a worsening condition. Blood pressure increases (not decreases) as a result of increased peripheral resistance. Increasing (not decreasing) edema would suggest a worsening condition. Trace levels to +1 proteinuria are acceptable levels. Higher levels would indicate a worsening condition.
CN: Health promotion and maintenance; CNS: None; CL: Application

38. 4. When the umbilical cord precedes the fetal presenting part, it's known as a prolapsed cord. Leaving the fingers in place and calling for assistance is the safest intervention for the fetus, as you'll need to keep the fetus off the cord to reduce cord compression. The nursing staff will contact the physician, and the client will probably need a cesarean delivery because of the risk of fetal demise with the fetus pressing against the cord during delivery. Placing the client in the semi-Fowler's position would increase the pressure of the fetus on the umbilical cord. Asking the client to push with the next contraction would be contraindicated, as it would also force the presenting part against the cord, causing severe bradycardia and possible fetal demise.
CN: Physiological integrity; CNS: Reduction of risk potential; CL: Application

39. 2. Monitoring fetal heart tones would be the first step because it's necessary to establish fetal well-being due to a possible placenta previa or abruptio placentae. Although an indwelling catheter may be placed, it isn't an early intervention. Performing a cervical examination would be contraindicated because any agitation of the cervix with a previa can result in hemorrhage and death for the mother or fetus. Preparing the client for a cesarean delivery may not be indicated. A sonogram will need to be performed to determine the cause of bleeding. If the diagnosis is a partial placenta previa, the client may still be able to deliver vaginally.
CN: Physiological integrity; CNS: Reduction of risk potential; CL: Application

40. A client in labor is receiving magnesium sulfate to treat hypertension of pregnancy. How should this drug be administered?
1. As a loading dose of 4 g in normal saline solution, followed by a continuous infusion of 1 to 2 g/hour
2. As a loading dose of 2 g in normal saline solution, followed by a continuous infusion of 2 g/hour
3. As a loading dose of 4 g in dextrose 5% in water (D_5W), followed by a continuous infusion of 1 to 2 g/hour
4. As a loading dose of 4 grams in D_5W, followed by a continuous infusion of 4 g/hour

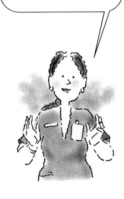

You're really "delivering" the right answers. Keep going!

40. 3. A loading dose of magnesium sulfate should be given as a 4-g bolus, followed by a continuous infusion of 1 to 2 g/hour in D_5W for maintenance. Magnesium sulfate shouldn't be administered in normal saline solution.

CN: Physiological integrity; CNS: Pharmacological and parenteral therapies; CL: Application

41. A multiparous client who has been in labor for 2 hours states that she feels the urge to move her bowels. How should the nurse respond?
1. Let the client get up to use the toilet.
2. Allow the client to use a bedpan.
3. Perform a pelvic examination.
4. Check the fetal heart rate (FHR).

41. 3. A complaint of rectal pressure usually indicates a low presenting fetal part, signaling imminent delivery. The nurse should perform a pelvic examination to assess the dilation of the cervix and station of the presenting fetal part. Don't let the client use the toilet or a bedpan before she's examined because she could deliver on the toilet or in the bedpan. Checking the FHR is important but comes after the nurse evaluates the client's complaint.

CN: Health promotion and maintenance; CNS: None; CL: Application

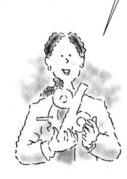

Your math skills are being tested on this one! You can do it!

42. The physician has ordered an I.V. of 5% dextrose in lactated Ringer's solution at 125 ml/hr. The I.V. tubing delivers 10 drops per ml. How many drops per minute should fall into the drip chamber?
1. 10 to 11
2. 12 to 13
3. 20 to 21
4. 22 to 24

42. 3. Multiply the number of milliliters to be infused (125) by the drop factor (10); $125 \times 10 = 1,250$. Then divide the answer by the number of minutes to run the infusion (60); $1,250 \div 60 = 20.83$, or 20 to 21 gtt/minute.

CN: Physiological integrity; CNS: Pharmacological and parenteral therapies; CL: Application

43. An amniotomy is performed on a client in labor. Following this procedure what is the priority nursing intervention?
1. Encourage the client to use breathing exercises as contractions increase.
2. Assess fetal heart tones.
3. Assist the client to ambulate to promote labor.
4. Position the client on her left side.

43. 2. The nurse's priority is to assess fetal heart tones. When the amniotic membrane is ruptured, the umbilical cord may enter the birth canal with the gush of fluid and the presenting part may cause cord compression. After amniotomy, contractions may intensify; however, helping the client with her breathing should be done after fetal well-being is assessed. Ambulation may also promote labor, but should only be done after fetal well-being is established. While the left lateral position enhances blood flow, it isn't a priority until fetal heart tones are assessed.

CN: Physiological integrity; CNS: Reduction of risk potential; CL: Application

CN: Client needs category   CNS: Client needs subcategory   CL: Cognitive level

44. The effectiveness of drug therapy for a client at 34 weeks' gestation with hypertension of pregnancy can be determined by which finding?
1. Absence of seizures
2. Weight gain of 4 lb (1.8 kg)/week
3. Blood pressure of 154/90 mm Hg
4. Urinary output of 25 ml/hour

45. A laboring client in the latent stage of labor begins complaining of pain in the epigastric area, blurred vision, and a headache. The nurse knows that which medication should be prepared for administration?
1. Terbutaline
2. Oxytocin (Pitocin)
3. Magnesium sulfate
4. Calcium gluconate

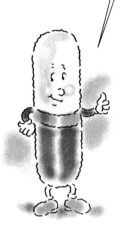

It's important to know how to measure a drug's effectiveness.

46. A nurse is assisting in monitoring a client in labor. Which monitoring data are indicative of fetal well-being?
1. Fetal heart rate of 145 to 155 beats/minute with 15-second accelerations to 160.
2. Fetal heart rate of 130 to 140 beats/minute with late decelerations to 110.
3. Fetal heart rate of 110 to 120 beats/minute with variable deceleration to 90.
4. Fetal heart rate of 165 to 175 beats/minute with late decelerations to 140.

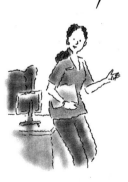

Remembering when different decelerations occur is important!

47. A nurse is examining a client in active labor who has had spontaneous rupture of the amniotic membrane and notes a protruding umbilical cord. What is the priority nursing action the nurse should take?
1. Push the umbilical cord into the uterus.
2. Place the client in Trendelenburg position.
3. Instruct the client to begin to push.
4. Wrap the cord in a dry sterile dressing.

44. 1. Therapeutic effects of drugs used to treat hypertension of pregnancy in a client at 34 weeks' gestation, such as magnesium sulfate, include an absence of seizures, a weight gain of 2 lb (0.9 kg)/week, a normal blood pressure, and a urinary output greater than 30 ml/hour.
CN: Physiological integrity; CNS: Pharmacological and parenteral therapies; CL: Analysis

45. 3. Magnesium sulfate is the drug of choice to treat hypertension of pregnancy because it reduces edema by causing a shift from the extracellular spaces into the intestines. It also depresses the central nervous system, which decreases the incidence of seizures. Terbutaline is a smooth-muscle relaxant used to relax the uterus. Oxytocin is the synthetic form of the pituitary hormone used to stimulate uterine contractions. Calcium gluconate is the antagonist for magnesium toxicity.
CN: Physiological integrity; CNS: Pharmacological and parenteral therapies; CL: Analysis

46. 1. Accelerations of up to 15 beats/minute above baseline for a duration of 15 seconds are signs of fetal well-being. Decelerations initiated 30 to 40 seconds after the onset of the contraction are termed late decelerations and are due to uteroplacental insufficiency from decreased blood flow during uterine contractions. Variable decelerations are an indication of cord compression. Variable decelerations can occur with or without contractions.
CN: Physiological integrity; CNS: Physiological adaptation; CL: Analysis

47. 2. A Trendelenburg or knee-chest position takes the weight of the fetus off the umbilical cord, allowing blood to flow. The cord should never be pushed back into the uterus, as this could damage the cord, obsruct the flow of blood through the cord to the fetus, or introduce infection into the uterus. The client shouldn't be instructed to push as she is only in active labor and emergency surgery may be necessary. The cord should be wrapped in a sterile saline soaked gauze.
CN: Physiological integrity; CNS: Reduction of risk potential; CL: Application

48. The first day of a client's last menstrual period (LMP) was October 10. Using Nägele's rule, what is the estimated date of delivery?
1. July 10
2. July 17
3. August 10
4. August 17

49. At 1 minute of life, a neonate is crying vigorously, has a heart rate of 98, is active with normal reflexes, and has a pink body and blue extremities. Which Apgar score would be correct for this neonate?
1. 6
2. 7
3. 8
4. 9

50. A client in labor suddenly sits upright, clutches her chest, and gasps for breath. Which laboratory finding indicates that the client's condition is worsening?
1. Increased fibrinogen level
2. Increased platelet count
3. Prolonged prothrombin time
4. Reduced partial thromboplastin time

51. Immediately after delivery, a nurse assesses the neonate's respiratory effort as slow. The neonate is actively moving but grimaces in response to stimulation. His fingers and toes are bluish, and his heart rate is 130 beats/minute. Which step should the nurse take next?
1. Tell the physician that the neonate appears abnormal.
2. Assign an Apgar score of 8.
3. Assign an Apgar score of 10.
4. Provide oxygen and stimulate the baby to cry.

Can you figure out this little one's estimated time of arrival?

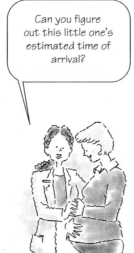

48. 2. After determining the first day of the LMP, the nurse would subtract 3 months and add 7 days. If the client's LMP was October 10, subtracting 3 months is July 10, and adding 7 days brings the date to July 17.
CN: Health promotion and maintenance; CNS: None; CL: Analysis

49. 3. Heart rate, respiratory effort, muscle tone, reflex irritability, and color are used to assess the Apgar score. Each of the signs is assigned a score of 0, 1, or 2. The highest possible score is 10. This neonate lost 1 point for a heart rate less than 100 beats/minute and 1 point for its acrocyanosis, a common finding in which the trunk is pink but the extremities are bluish.
CN: Health promotion and maintenance; CNS: None; CL: Analysis

50. 3. The client most likely has an amniotic fluid embolism. Disseminated intravascular coagulation is a life-threatening complication of this condition and is marked by a decreased platelet count and fibrinogen level, and a prolonged prothrombin time and partial thromboplastin time.
CN: Physiological integrity; CNS: Reduction of risk potential; CL: Analysis

51. 4. The nurse should stimulate the baby to cry, provide oxygen, and call the physician to evaluate reflex irritability. It would be inappropriate to tell the physician that the neonate appears abnormal. The neonate's Apgar score is 7. Of a maximum possible score of 10, the nurse deducts 1 point for acrocyanosis, 1 point for slow respiratory effort, and 1 point for the grimace (indicating reflex irritability).
CN: Safe, effective care environment; CNS: Management of care; CL: Application

CN: Client needs category   CNS: Client needs subcategory   CL: Cognitive level

52. A pregnant client has a total hemoglobin level of 9 g/dl. Which risk is <u>greatest</u> during the intrapartum period?
1. Small-for-gestational-age neonate
2. Fetal distress
3. Excessive postpartum bleeding
4. Shortness of breath

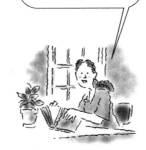

What do you think is the greatest risk?

52. 2. Fetal distress is more common in women with anemia than in the general non-anemic population. A small-for-gestational-age neonate and excessive postpartum bleeding are diagnosed after the intrapartum period. Shortness of breath occurs more commonly ante-partally; the risk for developing shortness of breath doesn't increase during the intrapartum period.
CN: Physiological integrity; CNS: Reduction of risk potential; CL: Application

53. Which is the <u>most common</u> and popular method for assessing fetal status throughout labor?
1. Fetal heart rate (FHR) auscultation using a stethoscope
2. FHR auscultation and recording using electronic fetal monitoring
3. Asking the client how she feels and whether the fetus is moving
4. Doing pelvic examinations to check the location of the fetal presenting part

53. 2. The most common and popular method for fetal assessment throughout labor is electronic monitoring, which records the FHR and maternal contractions and shows how the fetus reacts to the stress of contractions. Although FHR auscultation can be done with a stethoscope, it's less common because it requires advanced skills. Asking the client how she feels and whether the fetus is moving are important but don't provide specifics about fetal well-being. A pelvic examination reveals cervical dilation and fetal station but doesn't reveal fetal well-being.
CN: Health promotion and maintenance; CNS: None; CL: Analysis

54. Which finding in a client who is at 36 weeks' gestation indicates that premature rupture of the membranes has occurred?
1. Fernlike pattern when vaginal fluid dries on a glass slide
2. Nitrogen paper indicates acidic pH of fluid
3. Cervical dilation of 8 cm
4. Contractions occurring every 3 minutes

There are three main fetal presentations: Cephalic, breech, and shoulder.

54. 1. A fernlike pattern that forms when vaginal fluid is dried on a glass slide is a sign of ruptured membranes. Amniotic fluid is alkaline when tested with nitrogen paper. Cervical dilation and length of contractions don't indicate the condition of the membranes.
CN: Physiological integrity; CNS: Reduction of risk potential; CL: Application

55. The nurse is teaching an intrapartum client about fetal presentation. Which statement would be the most accurate?
1. Fetal body part that enters the maternal pelvis first
2. Relationship of the presenting part to the maternal pelvis
3. Relationship of the long axis of the fetus to the long axis of the mother
4. A classification according to the fetal part

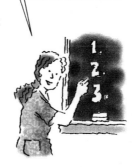

55. 1. Presentation is the fetal body part that enters the pelvis first; it's classified by the presenting part; the three main presentations are cephalic, breech, and shoulder. The relationship of the presenting fetal part to the maternal pelvis refers to fetal position. The relationship of the long axis of the fetus to the long axis of the mother refers to fetal lie; the three possible lies are longitudinal, transverse, and oblique.
CN: Physiological integrity; CNS: Physiological adaptation; CL: Application

56. A client with gestational diabetes has just delivered a 10-lb, 2-oz neonate at 39 weeks' gestation. Which priority nursing intervention should be included in the care plan?
1. Teach the mother about the nutritional needs of the neonate.
2. Obtain a serum neonatal glucose level.
3. Obtain a serum neonatal bilirubin level.
4. Prepare to administer insulin to the neonate.

56. 2. The priority nursing intervention is to monitor the neonate's serum glucose level due to the increased risk of hypoglycemia. During pregnancy the fetus secretes high levels of insulin to counteract the high maternal glucose levels. This elevated insulin secretion in the neonate can lead to severe hypoglycemia after birth. While it is important to discuss the neonate's nutritional needs with the mother, it isn't an immediate priority. The newborn of a mother with diabetes may develop hyperbilirubinemia, but not as quickly as hypoglycemia may develop. Since the neonate is at risk for hypoglycemia, insulin wouldn't be appropriate.
CN: Safe, effective care environment; CNS: Management of care; CL: Application

57. The nurse is caring for a client in labor. Which components of labor contractions would be the most accurate for the nurse to assess with this client?
1. Pelvic type, duration, and frequency
2. Contraction type and frequency, and pelvic type
3. Contraction duration, frequency, and intensity
4. Contraction type, duration, and intensity

57. 3. The three components of a contraction that the nurse must evaluate are the duration, frequency, and intensity of each contraction. Pelvic type has no bearing on contractions.
CN: Health promotion and maintenance; CNS: None; CL: Application

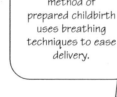

The Lamaze method of prepared childbirth uses breathing techniques to ease delivery.

58. A client in labor is using the Lamaze method of prepared childbirth. Her cervix is dilated 5 cm, with contractions occurring 2 to 3 minutes apart. The nurse should instruct the client to breathe at which level?
1. Level 1
2. Level 2
3. Level 3
4. Level 4

58. 2. Level 2 breathing techniques are useful when cervical dilation is between 4 and 6 cm. Level 1 breathing techniques are useful for early contractions; level 3 and level 4 breathing techniques are used in the transition stage of labor.
CN: Health promotion and maintenance; CNS: None; CL: Application

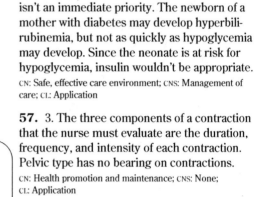

59. A client has received dinoprostone (Prostin E2) for cervical ripening. The nurse should assess her for which adverse drug effect?
1. Vomiting
2. Euphoria
3. Uterine inversion
4. Constipation

59. 1. Headache, nausea and vomiting, chills, fever, and hypertension are adverse effects of dinoprostone. Euphoria and uterine inversion are rare adverse effects of this drug. Diarrhea, not constipation, is a possible adverse effect.
CN: Physiological integrity; CNS: Pharmacological and parenteral therapies; CL: Analysis

60. A nurse is caring for a client with short, mild contractions and cervical dilation of 4 cm. Using an external fetal monitor, the nurse observes variable decelerations. Which action should the nurse take first?
1. Prepare for imminent delivery.
2. Place the client on her left side.
3. Administer oxygen by face mask.
4. Prepare the client for a still birth.

61. At 39 weeks' gestation, a primiparous client arrives at the labor-and-delivery unit complaining of lower back pain that started 6 hours ago. A pelvic examination reveals that her cervix is dilated 3 cm and 75% effaced. Which action would be appropriate for the nurse to take?
1. Instruct the client to push.
2. Determine the Apgar score.
3. Monitor the fetal heart rate.
4. Assess the lochia.

62. A nurse is assisting in monitoring a client who's receiving oxytocin (Pitocin) to induce labor. The nurse should be alert to which maternal adverse reactions? Select all that apply:
1. Hypertension
2. Jaundice
3. Dehydration
4. Fluid overload
5. Uterine tetany
6. Bradycardia

63. A client is admitted to the labor-and-delivery unit at 36 weeks' gestation. She has a history of cesarean delivery and complains of severe abdominal pain that started less than 1 hour earlier. When the nurse palpates tetanic contractions, the client again complains of severe pain. After the client vomits, she states that the pain is better and then passes out. Which nursing intervention takes the highest priority?
1. Assess the client's level of pain.
2. Place the client in a left lateral position.
3. Administer I.V. antibiotics.
4. Prepare the client for immediate surgery.

Don't give up now. Only three questions left!

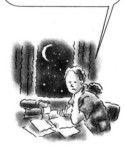

Keep up the good work!

60. 2. Variable decelerations in fetal heart rate are caused by compression of the umbilical cord. Typically, variable decelerations are corrected by placing the client in a left lateral position to alleviate cord pressure. Since variable decelerations are usually transient and correctable, the nurse wouldn't prepare for an imminent or still birth. If other measures have been ineffective in correcting the variable deceleration, oxygen may be administered.
CN: Physiological integrity; CNS: Reduction of risk potential; CL: Analysis

61. 3. This client is in the latent phase of the first stage of labor. The nurse should monitor the fetal heart in this stage and all stages of labor. Pushing is appropriate during the second stage of labor when the cervix is fully dilated. The nurse determines the Apgar score on the neonate immediately after delivery. During the fourth stage the nurse assesses the amount, color, and consistency of lochia.
CN: Health promotion and maintenance; CNS: None; CL: Application

62. 1, 4, 5. Adverse effects of oxytocin in the mother include hypertension, fluid overload, and uterine tetany. Oxytocin's antidiuretic effect increases renal reabsorption of water, leading to fluid overload, not dehydration. Jaundice and bradycardia are adverse effects that may occur in the neonate. Tachycardia, not bradycardia, is a maternal adverse effect.
CN: Physiological integrity; CNS: Pharmacology and parenteral therapies; CL: Application

63. 4. Uterine rupture is a medical emergency that may occur before or during labor. Signs and symptoms typically include abdominal pain that may ease after uterine rupture, vomiting, vaginal bleeding, hypovolemic shock, and fetal distress. The client should be prepared for immediate surgery to save her life and that of the fetus. While assessing and relieving pain are important interventions, they aren't priorities in this life-threatening situation. Placing the client in a left lateral position won't affect her condition. Antibiotics may be administered but aren't the highest priority in this situation.
CN: Safe, effective care environment; CNS: Management of care; CL: Application

64. Which illustration represents a right occiput posterior (ROP) fetal position?

1.
2.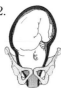

3.
4.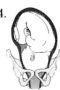

64. 1. Fetal positioning is determined by how the fetus presents in relation to the mother's pelvis, which is divided into four quadrants: right anterior, left anterior, right posterior, and left posterior. In a ROP position, the fetus' occiput points to the maternal right posterior quadrant. Option 2 shows a right occiput anterior (ROA) position, option 3 shows a left occiput posterior (LOP), and option 4 shows a left occiput anterior (LOA).

CN: Health promotion and maintenance; CNS: None; CL: Application

65. The nurse is evaluating an external fetal monitoring strip of a client in labor. What condition is the nurse concerned about?
1. Cephalopelvic disproportion
2. Oligohydramines
3. Uteroplacental insufficiency
4. Hydramnios

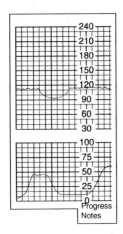

65. 3. This fetal monitoring strip illustrates a late deceleration. The decrease in fetal heart rate begins after the peak of the contraction and doesn't return to baseline until the contraction is over. Late decelerations are associated with uteroplacental insufficiency, shock, or fetal metabolic acidosis. Cephalopelvic disproportion may cause early not late decelerations early in labor. Oligohydramines (less than the normal amount of amniotic fluid) may be associated with variable decelerations. Hydramnios (excessive amniotic fluid) may be associated with uterine rupture.

CN: Physiological integrity; CNS: Reduction of risk potential; CL: Analysis

CN: Client needs category   CNS: Client needs subcategory   CL: Cognitive level

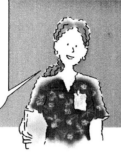

Chapter 9
Postpartum care

1. When completing the morning postpartum assessment, a nurse notices a client's perineal pad is completely saturated with lochia rubra. Which action should be the nurse's <u>first</u> response?
   1. Vigorously massage the fundus.
   2. Immediately call the physician.
   3. Have the charge nurse review the assessment.
   4. Ask the client when she last changed her perineal pad.

Question 1 is asking you what to do first! What a way to start!

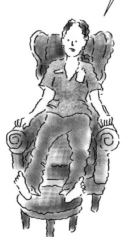

2. Which factor might result in a decreased supply of breast milk in a postpartum mother?
   1. Supplemental feedings with formula
   2. Maternal diet high in vitamin C
   3. An alcoholic drink
   4. Frequent feedings

Which of these options would promote comfort best?

3. Which intervention should be helpful to a breast-feeding mother with engorged breasts?
   1. Applying ice
   2. Applying a breast binder
   3. Teaching how to express her breasts in a warm shower
   4. Administering bromocriptine (Parlodel)

1. 4. If the morning assessment is done relatively early, it's possible that the client hasn't yet been to the bathroom, in which case her perineal pad may have been in place all night. Secondly, her lochia may have pooled during the night, resulting in a heavy flow in the morning. Vigorous massage of the fundus isn't recommended for heavy bleeding or hemorrhage. The nurse wouldn't want to call the physician unnecessarily. If the nurse were uncertain, it would be appropriate to have another qualified individual check the client but only after a complete assessment of the client's status.
CN: Safe, effective care environment; CNS: Management of care; CL: Analysis

2. 1. Routine formula supplementation may interfere with establishing an adequate milk volume because suckling by the baby at the breast stimulates prolactin production, the hormone responsible for milk production. Vitamin C levels haven't been shown to influence milk volume. One drink containing alcohol generally tends to relax the mother, facilitating letdown. Excessive consumption of alcohol may block letdown of milk to the infant, though supply isn't necessarily affected. Frequent feedings are likely to increase milk production.
CN: Health promotion and maintenance; CNS: None; CL: Application

3. 3. Teaching the client how to express her breasts in a warm shower aids with letdown and will give temporary relief. Ice can promote comfort by decreasing blood flow (vasoconstriction), numbing, and discouraging further letdown of milk; however, this is followed by a rebound reaction of more letting down once the ice is removed. Breast binders aren't effective in relieving the discomforts of engorgement. Bromocriptine is no longer indicated for lactation suppression.
CN: Physiological integrity; CNS: Basic care and comfort; CL: Application

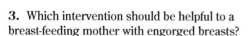
CN: Client needs category   CNS: Client needs subcategory   CL: Cognitive level

4. Which assessment should be performed routinely in the postpartum client?
1. Antibody screen
2. Babinski's reflex
3. Homans' sign
4. Patellar reflex

5. Which reason explains why Kegel exercises are advantageous to women after they deliver a child?
1. They assist with lochia removal.
2. They promote the return of normal bowel function.
3. They promote blood flow, allowing for healing and strengthening the musculature.
4. They assist the woman in burning calories for rapid postpartum weight loss.

If you know what Kegel exercises are, you should get question 5 correct easily.

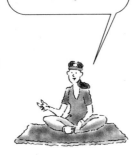

6. To detect pulmonary embolus in a client in the immediate postpartum period, a nurse should be alert to which symptoms?
1. Sudden dyspnea and chest pain
2. Chills and fever
3. Bradycardia and hypertension
4. Confusion and bradypnea

7. Which practice should a nurse recommend to a client who has had a cesarean delivery?
1. Frequent douching after she's discharged
2. Coughing and deep-breathing exercises
3. Sit-ups at 2 weeks postoperatively
4. Side-rolling exercises

4. 3. Homans' sign, or pain on dorsiflexion of the foot, may indicate deep vein thrombosis (DVT). Postpartum women are at increased risk of DVT because of changes in clotting mechanisms to control bleeding at delivery. An antibody screen wouldn't be classified as an assessment technique. Both Babinski's reflex and the patellar reflex need not be routinely assessed in the postpartum woman.
CN: Health promotion and maintenance; CNS: None; CL: Analysis

5. 3. Exercising the pubococcygeal muscle increases blood flow to the area. The increased blood flow brings oxygen and other nutrients to the perineal area to aid in healing. Additionally, these exercises help to strengthen the musculature, thereby decreasing the risk of future complications, such as incontinence and uterine prolapse. Performing Kegel exercises may assist with lochia removal but that isn't their main purpose. Bowel function isn't influenced by Kegel exercises. Kegel exercises don't expend sufficient energy to burn many calories.
CN: Health promotion and maintenance; CNS: None; CL: Analysis

6. 1. Signs of pulmonary embolus include sudden dyspnea and chest pain. Chills and fever signal an infection. The client with a pulmonary embolus would have tachycardia, hypotension, confusion, and tachypnea.
CN: Physiological integrity; CNS: Reduction of risk potential; CL: Analysis

7. 2. As for any postoperative client, coughing and deep-breathing exercises should be taught to keep the alveoli open and prevent infection. Frequent douching isn't recommended for women and is contraindicated in women who have just given birth. Sit-ups at 2 weeks postpartum could potentially damage the healing of the incision. Side-rolling exercises aren't an accepted medical practice.
CN: Physiological integrity; CNS: Reduction of risk potential; CL: Application

CN: Client needs category   CNS: Client needs subcategory   CL: Cognitive level

8. Which reason explains why a client might express disappointment after having a cesarean delivery instead of a vaginal delivery?
1. Cesarean deliveries cost more.
2. Depression is more common after a cesarean delivery.
3. The client is usually more fatigued after cesarean delivery.
4. The client may feel a loss for not having experienced a "normal" birth.

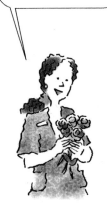

Remember to be sensitive to your postpartum client's needs.

9. Which finding is normal for a postpartum client who has experienced a vaginal birth?
1. Redness or swelling in the calves
2. A palpable uterine fundus beyond 10 days postpartum
3. Vaginal dryness after the lochial flow has ended
4. Dark red lochia for approximately 6 weeks after the birth

10. On completing a fundal assessment, the nurse notes the fundus is situated on the client's left abdomen. Which action is appropriate?
1. Ask the client to empty her bladder.
2. Straight catheterize the client immediately.
3. Call the client's primary health care provider for direction.
4. Straight catheterize the client for half of her urine volume.

11. A client who is positive for human immunodeficiency virus (HIV) tells a nurse she would like to breast-feed. Which is the best response by the nurse?
1. "Breast-feeding will help reduce the risk of hemorrhage."
2. "Breast milk is better than formula for the baby."
3. "Breast-feeding will help with bonding."
4. "Breast milk can transmit HIV to the baby."

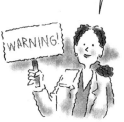

Make sure a client with HIV is aware of the risks of breast-feeding.

WARNING!

8. 4. Clients occasionally feel a loss after a cesarean delivery especially if it was unplanned. They may feel they're inadequate because they couldn't deliver their infant vaginally. The cost of cesarean delivery doesn't generally apply because the woman isn't directly responsible for payment. No conclusive studies support the theory that depression is more common after cesarean delivery when compared to vaginal delivery. Although clients are usually more fatigued after a cesarean delivery, fatigue hasn't been shown to cause feelings of disappointment over the method of delivery.
CN: Psychosocial integrity; CNS: None; CL: Analysis

9. 3. Vaginal dryness is a normal finding during the postpartum period due to hormonal changes. Redness or swelling in the calves may indicate thrombophlebitis. The fundus shouldn't be palpable beyond 10 days. Dark red lochia (indicating fresh bleeding) should only last 2 to 3 days postpartum.
CN: Health promotion and maintenance; CNS: None; CL: Application

10. 1. A full bladder may displace the uterine fundus to the left or right side of the abdomen. A straight catheterization is unnecessarily invasive if the woman can urinate on her own. Nursing interventions should be completed before notifying the primary health care provider in a nonemergency situation.
CN: Physiological integrity; CNS: Reduction of risk potential; CL: Application

11. 4. Since HIV can be transmitted to the baby through breast milk, the client shouldn't breast-feed. Breast-feeding does stimulate uterine contractions, but in this case, breast-feeding should be discouraged. It wouldn't be appropriate to tell a client who shouldn't breast-feed that breast milk is best for the baby. In this case, formula is best. The client should be shown other ways to bond with her baby, such as holding, playing, and talking to the baby.
CN: Physiologic integrity; CNS: Reduction of risk potential; CL: Analysis

12. A client had a spontaneous vaginal delivery after 18 hours of labor. Her excessive vaginal bleeding has now become a postpartum hemorrhage. <u>Immediate</u> nursing care of this client should include which intervention?
1. Avoiding massaging the uterus
2. Monitoring vital signs every hour
3. Placing the client in Trendelenburg's position
4. Elevating the head of the bed to increase blood flow

13. Which complication should a nurse assess for in a client with type 1 diabetes mellitus whose delivery was complicated by polyhydramnios and macrosomia?
1. Postpartum mastitis
2. Increased insulin needs
3. Postpartum hemorrhage
4. Gestational hypertension

14. The nurse is caring for a diabetic, postpartum client who has developed an infection. The nurse is aware that infections in diabetic clients tend to be more severe and can quickly lead to complications. For which complication should the nurse assess this client?
1. Anemia
2. Ketoacidosis
3. Respiratory acidosis
4. Respiratory alkalosis

15. Which client action should alert a nurse to a potential problem in a client with mastitis?
1. Breast-feeding every 6 hours
2. Breast-feeding on the affected breast first
3. Increasing daily fluid intake
4. Emptying the affected breast completely with each feeding

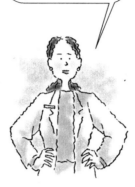

This question requires your immediate attention.

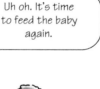

Uh oh. It's time to feed the baby again.

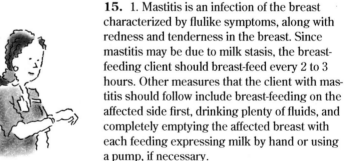

12. 3. The client should be placed in Trendelenburg's position to prevent or control hypovolemic shock. The uterus should be palpated to determine if it's contracting and should be massaged if it's boggy or not contracting. Vital signs should be monitored continuously, or at least every 10 to 15 minutes, until the client's condition stabilizes. The head of the bed shouldn't be elevated because this will further lower the blood pressure.
CN: Safe, effective care environment; CNS: Management of care; CL: Analysis

13. 3. The client is at risk for a postpartum hemorrhage from the overdistention of the uterus because of the extra amniotic fluid and the large baby. The uterus may not be able to contract as well as it would normally. The diabetic mother usually has decreased insulin needs for the first few days postpartum. Neither polyhydramnios nor macrosomia would increase the client's risk of mastitis or gestational hypertension.
CN: Physiological integrity; CNS: Reduction of risk potential; CL: Application

14. 2. Diabetic clients who become pregnant tend to become sicker and develop illnesses quicker than pregnant women without diabetes. Severe infections in diabetes can lead to diabetic ketoacidosis. Anemia, respiratory acidosis, and respiratory alkalosis aren't generally associated with infections in diabetic clients.
CN: Physiological integrity; CNS: Reduction of risk potential; CL: Analysis

15. 1. Mastitis is an infection of the breast characterized by flulike symptoms, along with redness and tenderness in the breast. Since mastitis may be due to milk stasis, the breast-feeding client should breast-feed every 2 to 3 hours. Other measures that the client with mastitis should follow include breast-feeding on the affected side first, drinking plenty of fluids, and completely emptying the affected breast with each feeding expressing milk by hand or using a pump, if necessary.
CN: Physiological integrity; CNS: Physiological adaptation; CL: Analysis

CN: Client needs category   CNS: Client needs subcategory   CL: Cognitive level

16. A nurse is assessing a client on the sixth postpartum day. Which condition requires prompt nursing action?
1. Blood loss in excess of 300 ml, occurring 24 hours to 6 weeks after delivery
2. Blood loss in excess of 500 ml, occurring 24 hours to 6 weeks after delivery
3. Blood loss in excess of 800 ml, occurring 24 hours to 6 weeks after delivery
4. Blood loss in excess of 1,000 ml, occurring 24 hours to 6 weeks after delivery

16. 2. Postpartum hemorrhage involves blood loss in excess of 500 ml. Most delayed postpartum hemorrhages occur between the fourth and ninth days postpartum. The most frequent causes of a delayed postpartum hemorrhage include retained placental fragments, intrauterine infection, and fibroids.
CN: Physiological integrity; CNS: Reduction of risk potential; CL: Application

17. Which assessment of the mother should be made in the <u>immediate</u> postpartum period (first 2 hours)?
1. Blood glucose level
2. Electrocardiogram (ECG)
3. Height of fundus
4. Stool test for occult blood

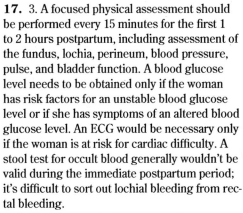

Question 17 requires your immediate attention.

17. 3. A focused physical assessment should be performed every 15 minutes for the first 1 to 2 hours postpartum, including assessment of the fundus, lochia, perineum, blood pressure, pulse, and bladder function. A blood glucose level needs to be obtained only if the woman has risk factors for an unstable blood glucose level or if she has symptoms of an altered blood glucose level. An ECG would be necessary only if the woman is at risk for cardiac difficulty. A stool test for occult blood generally wouldn't be valid during the immediate postpartum period; it's difficult to sort out lochial bleeding from rectal bleeding.
CN: Health promotion and maintenance; CNS: None; CL: Application

First things first! The word *initially* is a clue in this one.

18. In performing an assessment of a postpartum client 2 hours after delivery, a nurse notices heavy bleeding with large clots. Which response is most appropriate <u>initially</u>?
1. Massaging the fundus firmly
2. Performing bimanual compressions
3. Administering ergonovine (Ergotrate)
4. Notifying the physician

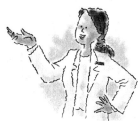

18. 1. Initial management of excessive postpartum bleeding is firm massage of the fundus along with a rapid infusion of oxytocin or lactated Ringer's solution. Bimanual compression is performed by a physician. Ergotrate should be used only if the bleeding doesn't respond to massage and oxytocin. The physician should be notified if the client doesn't respond to fundal massage, but other measures can be taken in the meantime.
CN: Safe, effective care environment; CNS: Management of care; CL: Analysis

19. A nurse is about to give a client with type 2 diabetes mellitus her insulin before breakfast on her first day postpartum. Which statement by the client indicates an understanding of insulin requirements immediately postpartum?
1. "I will need less insulin now than during my pregnancy."
2. "I will need more insulin now than during my pregnancy."
3. "I will need less insulin now than before I was pregnant."
4. "I will need more insulin now than before I was pregnant."

19. 3. Postpartum insulin requirements are usually significantly lower than prepregnancy requirements. Occasionally, clients may require little to no insulin during the first 24 to 48 hours postpartum.
CN: Physiological integrity; CNS: Reduction of risk potential; CL: Analysis

20. Which assessment finding in a postpartum client requires further nursing assessment?
1. Fundus at the umbilicus 1 hour postpartum
2. Fundus 3 cm below the umbilicus on postpartum day 3
3. Fundus not palpable in the abdomen at 2 weeks postpartum
4. Fundus slightly to right; 2 cm above umbilicus on postpartum day 2

21. Which condition should the nurse look for in a client's history that may explain an increase in the severity of afterpains?
1. Bottle-feeding
2. Diabetes
3. Multiple gestation
4. Primiparity

22. When giving a postpartum client self-care instructions, a nurse instructs her to report heavy or excessive bleeding. Which statement by the client indicates, she understands the nurse's instructions?
1. "I will call the doctor if I saturate a pad in 1 hour or less."
2. "I will call the doctor if I partially saturate a pad in 1 hour."
3. "I will call the doctor if I saturate a pad in 4 to 6 hours."
4. "I will call the doctor if I saturate a pad in 8 hours."

23. The nurse is assessing a postpartum client who has *lochia serosa* (old blood, serum, leukocytes, and tissue debris). When the client asks the nurse how long to expect this type of bleeding, the nurse's response should be?
1. Days 3 and 4 postpartum
2. Days 3 to 10 postpartum
3. Days 10 to 14 postpartum
4. Days 14 to 42 postpartum

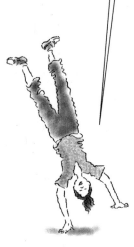

You're doing great! Keep up the good work!

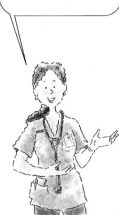

Remember: There are 3 types of lochia. Which type is this question referring to?

20. 4. A uterus that isn't midline or is above the umbilicus on postpartum day 2 might be caused by a full, distended bladder or a uterine infection, requiring further assessment by the nurse. Within the first 12 hours postpartum, the fundus usually is at or below the umbilicus. The fundus should descend approximately 1 cm/day, thereafter. The fundus shouldn't be palpated in the abdomen after day 10.
CN: Health promotion and maintenance; CNS: None; CL: Analysis

21. 3. Multiple gestation, breast-feeding, multiparity, and conditions that cause overdistention of the uterus will increase the intensity of afterpains. Bottle-feeding and diabetes aren't directly associated with increasing severity of afterpains, unless the client has delivered a macrosomic infant.
CN: Health promotion and maintenance; CNS: None; CL: Analysis

22. 1. Bleeding is considered heavy when a woman saturates a sanitary pad in 1 hour. Excessive bleeding occurs when a postpartum client saturates a pad in 15 minutes. Moderate bleeding occurs when the bleeding saturates less than 6″ (15 cm) of a pad in 1 hour.
CN: Health promotion and maintenance; CNS: None; CL: Application

23. 2. On the third and fourth postpartum days, the lochia becomes a pale pink or brown and contains old blood, serum, leukocytes, and tissue debris. This type of lochia usually lasts until postpartum day 10. Lochia rubra usually last for the first 3 to 4 days postpartum and consists of blood, decidua, and trophoblastic debris. Lochia alba, which contains leukocytes, decidua, epithelial cells, mucus, and bacteria, may continue for 2 to 6 weeks postpartum.
CN: Health promotion and maintenance; CNS: None; CL: Application

CN: Client needs category   CNS: Client needs subcategory   CL: Cognitive level

24. A client and her neonate have a blood incompatibility, and the neonate has had a positive direct Coombs' test. Which nursing intervention is appropriate?
1. Because the woman has been sensitized, give $Rh_0(D)$ immune globulin (RhoGAM).
2. Because the woman hasn't been sensitized, give RhoGAM.
3. Because the woman has been sensitized, don't give RhoGAM.
4. Because the woman hasn't been sensitized, don't give RhoGAM.

25. The nurse is teaching a client with newly-diagnosed mastitis about her condition. The nurse would inform the client that she <u>most likely</u> contracted the disorder from which organism?
1. *Escherichia coli (E. coli)*
2. Group beta-hemolytic streptococci (GBS)
3. *Staphylococcus aureus (S. aureus)*
4. *Staphylococcus pyogenes (S. pyogenes)*

26. A nurse should expect to observe which behavior in a client on the 4th postpartum day?
1. The client asks many questions about the baby's care.
2. The client wants to relate her birth experience.
3. The client asks the nurse to select her meals for her.
4. The client asks the nurse to help her bathe herself.

27. Which verbalization should be cause for concern to a nurse treating a postpartum client within a few days of delivery?
1. The client is nervous about taking the baby home.
2. The client feels empty since she delivered the baby.
3. The client would like to watch the nurse give the baby her first bath.
4. The client would like the nurse to take her baby to the nursery so she can sleep.

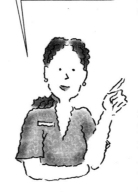

Blood incompatibility between a client and her neonate is serious business.

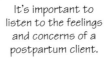

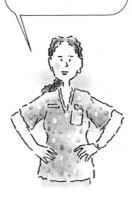

It's important to listen to the feelings and concerns of a postpartum client.

24. 3. A positive Coombs' test means that the Rh-negative woman is now producing antibodies to the Rh-positive blood of the neonate. RhoGAM shouldn't be given to a sensitized client because it won't be able to prevent antibody formation.
CN: Physiological integrity; CNS: Reduction of risk potential; CL: Analysis

25. 3. The most common cause of mastitis is *S. aureus*, transmitted from the neonate's mouth. Mastitis isn't harmful to the neonate. *E. coli*, GBS, and *S. pyogenes* aren't associated with mastitis. GBS infection is associated with neonatal sepsis and death.
CN: Health promotion and maintenance; CNS: None; CL: Analysis

26. 1. The taking-hold phase usually lasts from days 3 to 10 postpartum. During this stage, the mother strives for independence and autonomy; she also becomes curious and interested in the care of the baby and is most ready to learn. During the taking-in phase, which usually lasts 2 to 3 days, the mother is passive and dependent and expresses her own needs rather than the neonate's needs. During this taking-in phase, the client may ask the nurse to help her with self-care, wants to talk about the birth experience, and lets others make decisions for her.
CN: Psychosocial integrity; CNS: None; CL: Application

27. 2. A mother experiencing postpartum blues may say she feels empty now that the infant is no longer in her uterus. She may also verbalize that she feels unprotected now. Many first-time mothers are nervous about caring for their neonates by themselves after discharge. New mothers may want a demonstration before doing a task themselves. A client may want to get some uninterrupted sleep so she may ask that the baby be taken to the nursery.
CN: Psychosocial integrity; CNS: None; CL: Analysis

28. Which complication may be indicated by continuous seepage of blood from the vagina of a postpartum client, when palpation of the uterus reveals a firm uterus 1 cm below the umbilicus?
1. Retained placental fragments
2. Urinary tract infection (UTI)
3. Cervical laceration
4. Uterine atony

29. Which statement indicates to a nurse that a client needs further instruction on the use of anticoagulant therapy for deep vein thrombosis?
1. "I will continue to take my iron replacement therapy."
2. "I will take aspirin for headaches."
3. "I will avoid restrictive clothing."
4. "I will report shortness of breath immediately."

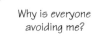

Why is everyone avoiding me?

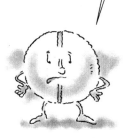

30. A pregnant client is very upset when she hears that her TORCH panel has returned positive. She is distraught and says, "This means the baby has HIV!" The nurse replies that the *H* in TORCH represents which of the following disorders?
1. Hemophilia
2. Hepatitis B virus
3. Herpes simplex virus
4. Human immunodeficiency virus

31. Which sign of grieving is <u>dysfunctional</u> in a client 3 days after a perinatal loss?
1. Lack of appetite
2. Denial of the death
3. Blaming herself
4. Frequent crying spells

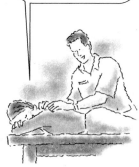

A good massage is just what the doctor, or in this case the nurse, ordered.

32. A nurse is assessing the fundus of a postpartum client and finds that the fundus is boggy. Which action should the nurse take first?
1. Prepare the client for surgery.
2. Administer blood replacement products.
3. Massage the fundus.
4. Administer methylergonovine, as ordered.

28. 3. Continuous seepage of blood may be due to cervical or vaginal lacerations if the uterus is firm and contracting. Retained placental fragments and uterine atony may cause subinvolution of the uterus, making it soft, boggy, and larger than expected. UTI won't cause vaginal bleeding, although hematuria may be present.
CN: Physiological integrity; CNS: Reduction of risk potential; CL: Application

29. 2. Discharge teaching should include informing the client to avoid salicylates, which may potentiate the effects of anticoagulant therapy. Iron won't affect anticoagulation therapy. Restrictive clothing should be avoided to prevent the recurrence of thrombophlebitis. Shortness of breath should be reported immediately because it may be a symptom of pulmonary embolism.
CN: Physiological integrity; CNS: Reduction of risk potential; CL: Analysis

30. 3. TORCH represents the following maternal infections: **T**oxoplasmosis; **O**thers, such as gonorrhea, syphilis, varicella, hepatitis, and human immunodeficiency virus; **R**ubella; Cytomegalovirus; and **H**erpes simplex virus. Hemophilia is a clotting disorder in which factors VII and X are deficient.
CN: Physiological integrity; CNS: Reduction of risk potential; CL: Application

31. 2. Denial of the perinatal loss is dysfunctional grieving in the client. Lack of appetite, blaming oneself, and frequent crying spells are part of a normal grieving process.
CN: Psychosocial integrity; CNS: None; CL: Application

32. 3. The nurse should first massage the boggy uterus to stimulate it to contract. The client may need surgery, but only if other measures fail to cause the uterus to contract and control bleeding. Blood replacement products may be given if the client has a significant blood loss. Methylergonovine may be ordered if massage fails to firm the uterus.
CN: Physiological integrity; CNS: Reduction of risk potential; CL: Analysis

CN: Client needs category   CNS: Client needs subcategory   CL: Cognitive level

33. An RH-positive client delivers a 6 lb, 10 oz neonate vaginally after 17 hours of labor. Which condition puts this client at risk for infection?
1. Length of labor
2. Maternal Rh status
3. Method of delivery
4. Size of the baby

34. When caring for a breast-feeding client who delivers by cesarean section, the nurse should teach the client to:
1. delay breast-feeding until 24 hours after delivery.
2. breast-feed frequently during the day and every 4 to 6 hours at night.
3. use the cradle hold position to avoid incisional discomfort.
4. use the football hold position to avoid incisional discomfort.

35. Which client behavior indicates an understanding of the nurse's teaching plan for breast-feeding?
1. The client washes her nipples with soap and water.
2. The client lets her nipples air-dry.
3. The client lets the baby attach to the nipple only.
4. The client pulls the baby off the nipple when feeding is done.

36. Which recommendation should be given to a client with mastitis who is concerned about breast-feeding her neonate?
1. She should stop breast-feeding until completing the antibiotic.
2. She should supplement feeding with formula until the infection resolves.
3. She shouldn't use analgesics because they aren't compatible with breast-feeding.
4. She should continue to breast-feed; mastitis won't infect the infant.

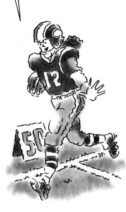

So that's what the coach meant by "holding."

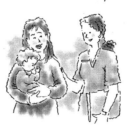

Mastitis shouldn't interfere with breast-feeding.

33. 1. A prolonged length of labor places the mother at increased risk for developing an infection. The average size of the baby, vaginal delivery, and Rh status of the client don't place the mother at increased risk.
CN: Physiological integrity; CNS: Physiological adaptation; CL: Analysis

34. 4. When breast-feeding after a cesarean delivery, the client should be encouraged to use the football hold to avoid incisional discomfort. Breast-feeding should be initiated as soon after birth as possible. The mother should be encouraged to breast-feed her infant every 2 to 3 hours throughout the night as well as during the day to increase the milk supply.
CN: Health promotion and maintenance; CNS: None; CL: Analysis

35. 2. The nipples should be allowed to air dry after breast-feeding to keep them dry and prevent irritation. Only water should be used to wash the nipples since soap removes natural oils and dries out the nipples. When breast-feeding, the baby should grasp both the nipple and areola. When the baby is done with a breast, the baby's grasp on the nipple should be released before removing the baby from the breast.
CN: Health promotion and maintenance; CNS: None; CL: Application

36. 4. The client with mastitis should be encouraged to continue breast-feeding while taking antibiotics for the infection. No supplemental feedings are necessary because breast-feeding doesn't need to be altered and actually encourages resolution of the infection. Analgesics are safe and should be administered as needed.
CN: Health promotion and maintenance; CNS: None; CL: Analysis

37. The nurse is assessing a 6-week-postpartum client in the obstetrician's office. In the exam room, the nurse asks the client how she's feeling. The client bursts into tears and reports she can barely get out of bed to dress, is crying most of the time, and feels like a failure. The nurse suspects the client is experiencing which of the following conditions?
 1. Postpartum blues
 2. Postpartum depression
 3. Postpartum neurosis
 4. Postpartum psychosis

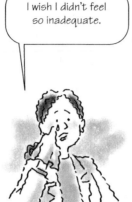

I wish I didn't feel so inadequate.

38. A client who is breast-feeding reports pain, redness, and swelling in her right breast. Which instruction should the nurse give the client?
 1. Wear a tight-fitting brassiere while breast-feeding.
 2. Breast-feeding should be stopped permanently.
 3. Continue antibiotic until pain, redness, and swelling subside.
 4. Apply moist heat compresses to the right breast.

39. A 6-week-postpartum client is being assessed by the nurse at the obstetrician's office. The nurse notes that the uterus is enlarged and soft and that the client is experiencing vaginal bleeding. The nurse suspects the client has which of the following conditions?
 1. Cervical laceration
 2. Clotting deficiency
 3. Perineal laceration
 4. Uterine subinvolution

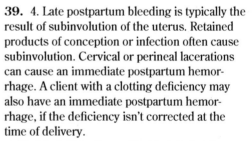

All I did was stand up, and I'm so light-headed!

40. A client needs to void 3 hours after a vaginal delivery. Which risk factor necessitates assisting her out of bed?
 1. Chest pain
 2. Breast engorgement
 3. Orthostatic hypotension
 4. Separation of episiotomy incision

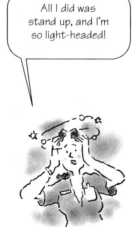

37. 2. Postpartum depression occurs in approximately 10% to 15% of all postpartum women. This depression is characterized by disabling feelings of inadequacy and an inability to cope that can last up to 3 years. The client is often tearful and despondent. The client with postpartum blues experiences crying and sadness, generally between 3 to 5 days postpartum, but this condition resolves itself quickly. Postpartum neurosis includes neurotic behavior during the initial 6 weeks after birth. Postpartum psychosis includes hallucinations, delusions, and phobias.
CN: Psychosocial integrity; CNS: None; CL: Application

38. 4. Moist heat compresses reduce inflammation and swelling of the affected area and relieves pain. The client shouldn't wear a tight or constrictive brassiere while breast-feeding to allow the milk to flow freely and empty the breast. There's no need to stop breast-feeding permanently. Antibiotics should be taken for the prescribed cause of therapy and shouldn't be stopped when symptoms subside.
CN: Health promotion and maintenance; CNS: None; CL: Application

39. 4. Late postpartum bleeding is typically the result of subinvolution of the uterus. Retained products of conception or infection often cause subinvolution. Cervical or perineal lacerations can cause an immediate postpartum hemorrhage. A client with a clotting deficiency may also have an immediate postpartum hemorrhage, if the deficiency isn't corrected at the time of delivery.
CN: Physiological integrity; CNS: Physiological adaptation; CL: Application

40. 3. The rapid decrease in intra-abdominal pressure occurring after birth causes splanchnic engorgement. The client is at risk for orthostatic hypotension when standing due to the blood pooling in this area. Breast engorgement is caused by vascular congestion in the breast before true lactation. The client shouldn't experience separation of the episiotomy incision or chest pain when standing.
CN: Health promotion and maintenance; CNS: None; CL: Analysis

41. Before giving a postpartum client the rubella vaccine, which fact should the nurse include in client teaching?
1. The vaccine is safe in clients with egg allergies.
2. Breast-feeding isn't compatible with the vaccine.
3. Transient arthralgia and rash are uncommon adverse effects.
4. The client should avoid getting pregnant for 3 months after the vaccination because the vaccine has teratogenic effects.

42. The nurse is caring for a postpartum client who develops preeclampsia. Which medication should the nurse expect to administer?
1. Diazepam (Valium)
2. Hydralazine
3. Magnesium sulfate
4. Nifedipine (Procardia)

43. Which complication is associated with magnesium sulfate therapy?
1. Hypotension
2. Postpartum depression
3. Postpartum hemorrhage
4. Uterine infection

44. Which intervention should be included in the plan of care for a client with an episiotomy on the third postpartum day?
1. Apply ice to the perineum.
2. Encourage the use of sitz baths.
3. Avoid tightening the pelvic muscles.
4. Massage the perineal area.

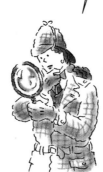

Don't lose your focus.

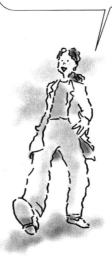

You're making great strides. Keep going!

41. 4. The client must understand that she must not become pregnant for 2 to 3 months after the vaccination because of its potential teratogenic effects. The rubella vaccine is made from duck eggs so an allergic reaction may occur in clients with egg allergies. The virus isn't transmitted into the breast milk, so clients may continue to breast-feed after vaccination. Transient arthralgia and rash are common adverse effects of the vaccine.
CN: Health promotion and maintenance; CNS: None; CL: Application

42. 3. Magnesium sulfate is commonly used in the treatment of preeclampsia to prevent seizures. It also produces a smooth muscle depression effect, which can lower blood pressure. Diazepam may also be given for seizure activity. Nifedipine and hydralazine are used for severely hypertensive preeclamptic women.
CN: Physiological integrity; CNS: Pharmacological and parenteral therapies; CL: Application

43. 3. Because magnesium sulfate relaxes smooth muscle, the uterus should be assessed for uterine atony, which would increase the risk of postpartum hemorrhage. Postpartum depression and uterine infection aren't associated with magnesium sulfate therapy. Magnesium sulfate is considered more of an anticonvulsant than an antihypertensive.
CN: Physiological integrity; CNS: Pharmacological and parenteral therapies; CL: Comprehension

44. 2. A sitz bath reduces inflammation and relaxes the perineum, promoting healing and reducing discomfort. Ice should only be used for the first 24 hours following delivery. Kegel exercises, which involve tightening and relaxing the pelvic muscles, improve circulation and reduce edema. Massaging the perineum may disrupt the suture line and cause more pain.
CN: Physiological integrity; CNS: Physiological adaptation; CL: Analysis

45. Which response is most appropriate for a mother with diabetes who wants to breast-feed but is concerned about the effects of breast-feeding on her health?

1. Mothers with diabetes who breast-feed have a hard time controlling their insulin needs.
2. Mothers with diabetes shouldn't breast-feed because of potential complications.
3. Mothers with diabetes shouldn't breast-feed; insulin requirements are doubled.
4. Mothers with diabetes may breast-feed; insulin requirements may decrease from breast-feeding.

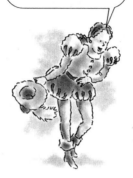

To breast-feed or not to breast-feed, that is the question.

46. Which activity by a client indicates that a nurse's teaching about perineal care has been effective?

1. The client uses a spray bottle to cleanse the perineum after urination and bowel movements.
2. The client wipes the perineum from back to front after urinating or a bowel movement.
3. The client douches after urination or a bowel movement.
4. The client changes perineal pads three times a day.

47. Which factor puts a multiparous client on her first postpartum day at risk for developing hemorrhage?

1. Hemoglobin level of 12 g/dl
2. Uterine atony
3. Thrombophlebitis
4. Moderate amount of lochia rubra

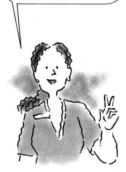

Remember, when you're dealing with a postpartum client, you've got two clients to think about.

48. On the first postpartum night, a client requests that her baby be sent back to the nursery so she can get some sleep. The client is most likely in which phase?

1. Depression phase
2. Letting-go phase
3. Taking-hold phase
4. Taking-in phase

45. 4. Breast-feeding has an antidiabetogenic effect. Insulin needs are decreased because carbohydrates are used in milk production. Breast-feeding mothers are at a higher risk of hypoglycemia in the first postpartum days after birth because the glucose levels are lower. Mothers with diabetes should be encouraged to breast-feed.
CN: Physiological integrity; CNS: Pharmacological and parenteral therapies; CL: Application

46. 1. The client should cleanse the perineal area after urinating or a bowel movement using a spray or peri-bottle. The client should wipe from front to back after urination or a bowel movement to avoid contaminating the perineal area. Perineal pads should be changed when they are soiled to keep the perineum clean.
CN: Health promotion and maintenance; CNS: None; CL: Application

47. 2. Multiparous women often experience a loss of uterine tone due to frequent distentions of the uterus from past pregnancies. As a result, this client is also at higher risk for hemorrhage. Thrombophlebitis doesn't increase the risk of hemorrhage during the postpartum period. The hemoglobin level and lochia flow are within acceptable limits.
CN: Health promotion and maintenance; CNS: None; CL: Analysis

48. 4. The taking-in phase occurs in the first 24 hours after birth. The mother is concerned with her own needs and requires support from staff and relatives. The depression phase isn't an appropriate answer. The letting-go phase begins several weeks later, when the mother incorporates the new infant into the family unit. The taking-hold phase occurs when the mother is ready to take responsibility for her care as well as her infant's care.
CN: Health promotion and maintenance; CNS: None; CL: Analysis

CN: Client needs category   CNS: Client needs subcategory   CL: Cognitive level

49. Four clients each gave birth 12 hours ago. Which one would most likely suffer complications after birth?
1. Gravida 2 Para 2002, cesarean birth, incisional site intact, hemoglobin level 9.8 g/dl
2. Gravida 2 Para 1011, cesarean birth, incisional site intact, pulse 84 beats/minute
3. Gravida 1 Para 1001, vaginal delivery, midline episiotomy, temperature 99.8° F (37.7° C)
4. Gravida 1 Para 1001, vaginal delivery, ruptured membranes 10 hours before delivery

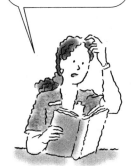

Which client is at the greatest risk for complications?

50. Which statement by a client shows she understands how to prevent breast engorgement while breast-feeding?
1. "I will apply moist heat to my breasts three times a day."
2. "I will breast-feed every 1 to 3 hours."
3. "I will use a breast pump to obtain milk for feedings."
4. "I will wear a tight bra continually."

51. A client has delivered twins. Which intervention would be most important for a nurse to perform?
1. Assess fundal tone and lochia flow.
2. Apply a cold pack to the perineal area.
3. Administer analgesics, as ordered.
4. Encourage voiding by offering the bedpan.

Question 52 is looking for a *normal* response.

52. Which physiological response is considered normal in the early postpartum period?
1. Urinary urgency and dysuria
2. Rapid diuresis
3. Decrease in blood pressure
4. Increased motility of the GI system

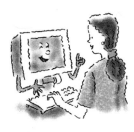

49. 1. Women who are anemic in pregnancy (defined as a hemoglobin < 10 g/dl) may experience more complications, such as poor wound healing and inability to tolerate activity. The vital signs in answers 2 and 3 are within normal limits. Dehydration can cause a slightly elevated temperature. Women whose membranes are ruptured more than 24 hours before birth are more prone to developing chorioamnionitis.
CN: Health promotion and maintenance; CNS: None; CL: Analysis

50. 2. Frequent breast-feeding empties the breast, decreasing the risk of engorgement. Moist heat can stimulate the let-down reflex, leading to engorgement. A breast pump isn't necessary if a baby is able to breast-feed regularly. A tight brassiere may prevent the breasts from emptying completely when breast-feeding, increasing the risk of engorgement.
CN: Health promotion and maintenance; CNS: None; CL: Application

51. 1. Women who deliver twins are at a higher risk for postpartum hemorrhage due to overdistention of the uterus, which causes uterine atony. Assessing fundal tone and lochia flow helps to determine risks for hemorrhage. Applying cold packs to the perineum, administering analgesics as ordered, and offering the bedpan are all significant nursing interventions but not as important as preventing postpartum hemorrhage.
CN: Health promotion and maintenance; CNS: None; CL: Analysis

52. 2. In the early postpartum period, there's an increase in the glomerular filtration rate and a drop in progesterone levels, which result in rapid diuresis. There should be no urinary urgency, though a woman may feel anxious about voiding. There's minimal change in blood pressure following childbirth, and a residual decrease in GI motility.
CN: Physiological integrity; CNS: Physiological adaptation; CL: Application

53. During the third postpartum day, which observation about a client should the nurse be <u>most likely</u> to make?
1. The client appears interested in learning more about neonatal care.
2. The client talks a lot about her birth experience.
3. The client sleeps whenever the neonate isn't present.
4. The client requests help in choosing a name for the neonate.

54. Which circumstance is most likely to cause uterine atony and lead to postpartum hemorrhage?
1. Hypertension
2. Cervical and vaginal tears
3. Urine retention
4. Endometritis

55. Which assessment requires immediate action by a nurse in a client 22 hours following a cesarean delivery?
1. Heart rate of 132 beats/minute and blood pressure of 84/60 mm Hg
2. Oral temperature of 100.2° F
3. A gush of blood from the vagina when the client stands up
4. Complaints of abdominal pain and cramping

56. Which percentage of postpartum clients experiences "postpartum blues"?
1. 20% to 25%
2. 50% to 80%
3. 30% to 45%
4. 100%

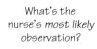

What's the nurse's most likely observation?

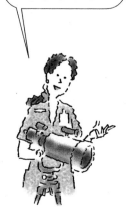

Have you ever heard the postpartum blues?

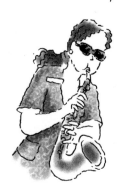

53. 1. By the third postpartum day, the client should be in the taking-hold phase, in which the new mother strives for independence and is eager for her neonate. The other options describe the phase in which the mother relives her birth experience.
CN: Health promotion and maintenance; CNS: None; CL: Analysis

54. 3. Urine retention causes a distended bladder to displace the uterus above the umbilicus and to the side, which prevents the uterus from contracting. The uterus needs to remain contracted if bleeding is to stay within normal limits. Cervical and vaginal tears can cause postpartum hemorrhage but are less common occurrences in the postpartum period. Maternal hypertension and endometritis don't cause postpartum hemorrhage.
CN: Health promotion and maintenance; CNS: None; CL: Application

55. 1. Tachycardia (heart rate of 132 beats/minute) and hypotension (blood pressure of 84/60 mm Hg) may be a sign of hemorrhage. An oral temperature of 100.2° F may be due to dehydration, when it occurs on the first postpartum day. A gush of blood from the vagina when a client stands is a normal finding on the first postpartum day. Complaints of abdominal pain and cramping are expected following cesarean delivery.
CN: Physiological integrity; CNS: Reduction of risk potential; CL: Application

56. 2. "Postpartum blues"—a transient mood alteration that arises during the first 3 weeks postpartum and is typically self-limiting—affects 50% to 80% of postpartum clients. A more severe mood alteration, seen in approximately 20% of clients, involves changes that occur within a few days after delivery and may last for a few days to more than 1 year.
CN: Psychosocial integrity; CNS: None; CL: Application

CN: Client needs category   CNS: Client needs subcategory   CL: Cognitive level

57. When performing a <u>comprehensive</u> fundal check during a postpartum assessment, a nurse evaluates which fundal state?
1. Fundal consistency, location, and height
2. Fundal consistency and height
3. Fundal location and potential fundal distention
4. Fundal location and height

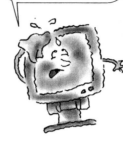

Don't sweat it! You're almost there!

57. 1. A comprehensive fundal check includes evaluation of fundal consistency, height, and location. Normal results are a firm fundus that's at the correct height for the postpartum day and located in the center of the pelvis. Options 2, 3, and 4 don't reflect a comprehensive fundal check because they're missing valuable components.
CN: Physiological integrity; CNS: Physiological adaptation; CL: Analysis

58. A nurse is performing an assessment on a postpartum client. The assessment reveals that the fundus is firm. This data indicates which condition?
1. A firm tumor at the top of the uterus
2. Contraction of the uterus
3. Continuing labor contractions
4. Bladder distention

58. 2. A firm postpartum fundus means that the uterus has contracted and is constricting blood vessels, thereby decreasing lochial flow. A uterine tumor doesn't necessarily cause a firm fundus. The client wouldn't experience labor contractions during the postpartum period. Bladder distention restricts the uterus from contracting downward, resulting in a soft, boggy uterus and increased vaginal bleeding.
CN: Physiological integrity; CNS: Physiological adaptation; CL: Analysis

59. A primipara who is Rho(D)-negative has just given birth to an Rh-positive baby. Which <u>priority</u> nursing intervention should be included in the plan of care?
1. Administer $Rh_0(D)$ immune globulin to the neonate within 3 days.
2. Administer $Rh_0(D)$ immune globulin to the client within 3 days.
3. Administer $Rh_0(D)$ immune globulin to the client at her first postpartum visit in 6 weeks.
4. Administer $Rh_0(D)$ immune globulin to the neonate at the first well-baby visit.

Discharge teaching is important. Which instruction should you include for your clients with DVT?

59. 2. Administering $Rh_0(D)$ immune globulin to the client within 72 hours of delivery prevents antibodies from forming that can destroy fetal blood cells in the next pregnancy. $Rh_0(D)$ immune globulin isn't given to the baby. The client shouldn't wait 6 weeks to receive $Rh_0(D)$ immune globulin as antibodies will already have formed.
CN: Safe, effective care environment; CNS: Management of care; CL: Application

60. A postpartum client is receiving anticoagulant therapy for deep vein thrombophlebitis. Discharge teaching should include which instruction?
1. Avoid iron replacement therapy.
2. Wear a girdle and knee-high stockings whenever possible.
3. Avoid over-the-counter salicylates.
4. Be aware that shortness of breath is a common adverse effect of anticoagulants.

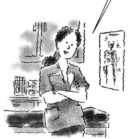

60. 3. Discharge teaching should include an instruction to avoid salicylates, which may magnify the effects of anticoagulant therapy. Iron doesn't affect anticoagulant therapy. The client should avoid restrictive clothing to prevent recurrence of thrombophlebitis. She should report shortness of breath immediately because it may indicate pulmonary embolus.
CN: Health promotion and maintenance; CNS: Reduction of risk potential; CL: Application

61. For a breast-feeding client on the fourth postpartum day, which breast examination findings are normal?
 1. Soft, nontender breasts
 2. Engorged breasts with inflamed, radiating areas that are sore to the touch
 3. Slightly tender, cracked nipples; slightly firm, nontender breasts; transitional milk
 4. Tender, intact nipples; firm, tender breasts; transitional milk

62. Which client statement should alert the nurse to a potential problem in a breast-feeding primiparous client?
 1. "I will consume an additional 500 calories/day."
 2. "I will increase my intake of protein."
 3. "I will limit my fluid intake."
 4. "I will eat foods high in vitamins and minerals."

63. A nurse is teaching a breast-feeding primiparous client how to prevent sore nipples. Which client statement indicates the need for further instruction?
 1. "I should breast-feed for only 3 to 4 minutes at a time until my milk flow is established."
 2. "I should position the baby properly during feedings."
 3. "I should pull the baby gently away from my nipple after the feeding."
 4. "I should prevent the baby from feeding after my breast has been emptied."

64. A client is 2 days postpartum and is talking with her nurse about the bleeding she's having, asking, "Will it always be so heavy?" Which statement by the nurse would be the <u>most accurate</u>?
 1. "This is lochia alba and will last 4 weeks."
 2. "This is lochia serosa and will last 2 days."
 3. "This is lochia rubra and will last 3–4 days."
 4. "This is your menstrual cycle and it will last 6 weeks."

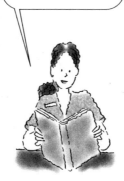

I need to determine which findings are normal for this client.

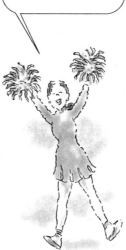

Only 7 more questions to go!

61. 4. Tender, intact nipples; firm, tender breasts; and transitional milk are normal in a breast-feeding client on the fourth postpartum day. Engorged, inflamed breasts signal mastitis. Tender, cracked nipples aren't a normal finding; they require intervention and client teaching to help the nipples heal and help the client avoid the problem in the future.
CN: Physiological integrity; CNS: Physiological adaptation; CL: Application

62. 3. A breast-feeding client who states that fluid intake should be limited should alert the nurse that more education is needed. Increased fluids are needed for milk production. The breast-feeding client should consume an additional 500 calories/day, increase protein intake, and eat foods high in vitamins and minerals.
CN: Health promotion and maintenance; CNS: None; CL: Application

63. 1. In some cases, it takes 7 minutes for the letdown reflex to cause milk to fill the breast. The other answers indicate that the client understands the nurse's instructions.
CN: Physiological integrity; CNS: Reduction of risk potential; CL: Application

64. 3. Lochia rubra, which is made up of blood, mucus, and tissue debris, lasts 3–4 days. Lochia serosa, which consists of blood, mucus, and leukocytes, lasts from day 3 to day 10 postpartum. Lochia alba, which consists largely of mucus, lasts from day 10 to day 14 postpartum. Lochia alba may last up to 6 weeks postpartum. Postpartum bleeding is not the menstrual cycle.
CN: Physiological integrity; CNS: Physiological adaptation; CL: Application

CN: Client needs category   CNS: Client needs subcategory   CL: Cognitive level

65. On examining a client who gave birth 3 hours ago, the nurse finds that the client has completely saturated a perineal pad within 15 minutes. Which actions should the nurse take? Select all that apply:

1. Begin an IV infusion of lactated Ringer's solution.
2. Assess the client's vital signs.
3. Palpate the client's fundus.
4. Place the client in high Fowler's position.
5. Administer a pain medication.

65. 2, 3. Assessing vital signs provides information about the client's circulatory status and identifies significant changes to report to the physician. By palpating the client's fundus, the nurse also gains valuable assessment data. A boggy uterus may lead to excessive bleeding. Starting an IV infusion requires a physician's order. Placing the client in high Fowler's position may lower blood pressure and be harmful to the client. Administration of a pain medication doesn't address the current problem.

CN: Physiological integrity; CNS: Reduction of risk potential; CL: Application

66. Which characteristic of lochia should a nurse expect in a client two weeks postpartum?

1. It's creamy white to brown and may have a stale odor.
2. It's creamy white to brown, contains decidual cells, and may have a stale odor.
3. It's brown to red, contains tissue fragments, and may have an odor.
4. It's brown to red and contains decidual cells and leukocytes.

66. 2. Lochia alba occurs from one to three weeks postpartum. Lochia alba is creamy white to brown, contains decidual cells, and may have a stale odor. It also contains leukocytes. Lochia alba shouldn't contain tissue fragments or have a foul odor.

CN: Physiological integrity; CNS: Physiological adaptation; CL: Application

67. In a client one week postpartum with retained placental fragments, which finding should alert a nurse of a common complication?

1. Puerperal infection
2. Postpartum depression
3. Postpartum hemorrhage
4. Uterine subinvolution

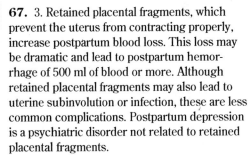

Stay with it! Just a few more to go!

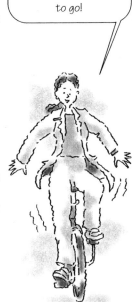

67. 3. Retained placental fragments, which prevent the uterus from contracting properly, increase postpartum blood loss. This loss may be dramatic and lead to postpartum hemorrhage of 500 ml of blood or more. Although retained placental fragments may also lead to uterine subinvolution or infection, these are less common complications. Postpartum depression is a psychiatric disorder not related to retained placental fragments.

CN: Health promotion and maintenance; CNS: None; CL: Application

68. The nurse is assisting in developing a care plan for a client who had an episiotomy. Which interventions would be included for the nursing diagnosis *Acute pain related to perineal sutures?* Select all that apply:

1. Apply an ice pack intermittently to the perineal area for 3 days.
2. Avoid the use of topical pain gels.
3. Administer sitz baths three to four times per day.
4. Encourage the client to do Kegel exercises.
5. Limit the number of times the perineal pad is changed.

68. 3, 4. Sitz baths help decrease inflammation and tension in the perineal area. Kegel exercises improve circulation to the area and help reduce edema. Ice packs should be applied to the perineum for the first 24 hours only; after that time, heat should be used. Topical pain gels should be applied to the suture area to reduce discomfort, as ordered. The perineal pad should be changed frequently to prevent irritation caused by the discharge.

CN: Physiological integrity; CNS: Basic care and comfort; CL: Application

69. A nurse is palpating the uterine fundus of a client who delivered a baby 8 hours ago. At what level in the abdomen would the nurse expect to feel the fundus?

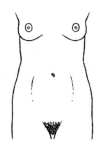

70. A mother with a past history of varicose veins has just delivered her first baby. A nurse suspects that the mother has developed pulmonary embolus. Which of the data below would lead to this nursing judgment? Select all that apply:
1. Sudden dyspnea
2. Chills, fever
3. Diaphoresis
4. Bradycardia
5. Confusion

71. A nurse observes several interactions between a mother and her neonate son. Which maternal behaviors should the nurse identify as evidence of mother-infant attachment? Select all that apply:
1. Talks and coos to her son.
2. Cuddles her son close to her.
3. Doesn't make eye contact with her son.
4. Requests that the nurse take the baby to the nursery for feedings.
5. Encourages the father to hold the baby.
6. Takes a nap when the baby is sleeping.

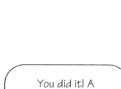

You did it! A star is born (no pun intended)!

69. The uterus should be felt at the level of the umbilicus from 1 hour after birth and for about the next 24 hours.
CN: Physiological integrity;
CNS: Reduction of risk potential;
CL: Application

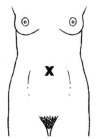

70. 1, 3, 5. Sudden dyspnea along with diaphoresis and confusion are classic symptoms that develop when a thrombus (stationary blood clot) from a varicose vein becomes an embolus (moving clot) that lodges in the pulmonary circulation. Chills and fever would indicate infection. A client with an embolus usually develops tachycardia.
CN: Physiological integrity; CNS: Physiological adaptation;
CL: Analysis

71. 1, 2. Talking, cooing, and cuddling with her son are positive signs of mother-infant attachment. Avoiding eye contact is a non-bonding behavior. Eye contact, touching, and speaking help establish attachment with a neonate. Feeding a neonate is an important role of a new mother and facilitates attachment. Encouraging the father to hold the neonate will facilitate attachment. Resting while the neonate is sleeping will conserve needed energy and allow the mother to be alert.
CN: Psychosocial integrity; CNS: None; CL: Analysis

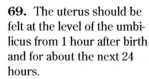

CN: Client needs category   CNS: Client needs subcategory   CL: Cognitive level

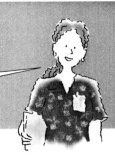

Neonates depend on you for *everything*. Let's show 'em you've got what it takes for neonatal care!

1. A client has given birth to a preterm male neonate. The client tells the nurse that she still wants to breast-feed her neonate. The nurse should explain to the mother that:
  1. breast milk contains antibodies that help protect her neonate.
  2. commercial formula will provide better nutrition for the neonate.
  3. breast-feeding can be started when the neonate is ready for discharge.
  4. the neonate will be less likely to develop an infection on commercial formula.

2. The parents of a neonate admitted to the NICU ask why the physician has ordered surfactant therapy. Which statement would be most accurate for parent education?
  1. Surfactant will help regulate the baby's breathing pattern.
  2. Surfactant helps clear mucus and fluid from the respiratory system to make breathing easier.
  3. Surfactant helps mature the upper airways to make breathing easier.
  4. Surfactant helps in keeping the lungs expanded after the baby starts breathing on its own.

3. While assessing a 2-hour-old neonate, a nurse observes the neonate to have acrocyanosis. Which nursing action should be performed initially?
  1. Activate the code blue or emergency system.
  2. Do nothing because acrocyanosis is normal in the neonate.
  3. Immediately take the neonate's temperature according to facility policy.
  4. Notify the physician of the need for a cardiac consult.

You need to keep the parents informed of the whats and whys of their baby's care.

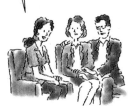

What do you need to do first?

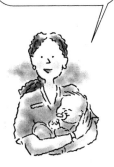

1. 1. Studies have proven that breast milk provides preterm neonates with better protection from infection, such as necrotizing enterocolitis, because of the antibodies contained in breast milk. Commercial formula doesn't provide any better nutrition than breast milk. Breast milk feedings can be started as soon as the neonate is stable. The neonate is more likely to develop infections when fed formula rather than breast milk.
CN: Health promotion and maintenance; CNS: None; CL: Application

2. 4. Surfactant works by reducing surface tension in the lung. It allows the lung to remain slightly expanded, decreasing the amount of work required for inspiration. Surfactant hasn't been shown to influence upper airway maturation, regulate the neonate's breathing pattern or clear the respiratory tract.
CN: Physiological integrity; CNS: Pharmacological and parental therapies; CL: Application

3. 2. Acrocyanosis, or bluish discoloration of the hands and feet in the neonate (also called *peripheral cyanosis*), is a normal finding and shouldn't last more than 24 hours after birth. The other choices are inappropriate.
CN: Physiological integrity; CNS: Physiological adaptation; CL: Application

CN: Client needs category   CNS: Client needs subcategory   CL: Cognitive level

4. When teaching parents of a neonate the proper position for the neonate's sleep, a nurse stresses the importance of placing the neonate on his back to reduce the risk of which of the following?
  1. Aspiration
  2. Sudden infant death syndrome (SIDS)
  3. Suffocation
  4. Gastroesophageal reflux (GER)

5. A nurse is caring for a client with gestational diabetes. Which complication is the neonate most at risk of developing?
  1. Anemia
  2. Hypoglycemia
  3. Nitrogen loss
  4. Thrombosis

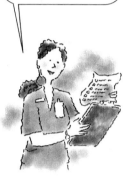

Knowing the risk factors can help guide your assessment.

6. Which complication is common in neonates who receive prolonged mechanical ventilation at birth?
  1. Bronchopulmonary dysplasia
  2. Esophageal atresia
  3. Hydrocephalus
  4. Renal failure

7. When performing neonatal assessment, which is the <u>best</u> indication of adequate hydration?
  1. Soft, smooth skin
  2. A sunken fontanel
  3. Bradycardia
  4. No urine output in the first 24 hours of life

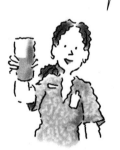

Here's to you! You're the best!!

4. 2. Supine positioning is recommended to reduce the risk of SIDS in infancy. The risk of aspiration is slightly increased with the supine position. Suffocation would be less likely with an infant supine than prone, and the position for GER requires the head of the bed to be elevated.
CN: Health promotion and maintenance; CNS: None; CL: Application

5. 2. Neonates of mothers with diabetes are at risk for hypoglycemia due to increased insulin levels. During gestation, an increased amount of glucose is transferred to the fetus through the placenta. The neonate's liver can't initially adjust to the changing glucose levels after birth. This may result in an overabundance of insulin in the neonate, resulting in hypoglycemia. Neonates of mothers with diabetes aren't at increased risk for anemia, nitrogen loss, or thrombosis.
CN: Physiological integrity; CNS: Physiological adaptation; CL: Analysis

6. 1. Bronchopulmonary dysplasia commonly results from the high pressures that must sometimes be used to maintain adequate oxygenation. Esophageal atresia, a structural defect in which the esophagus and trachea communicate with each other, doesn't relate to mechanical ventilation. Hydrocephalus and renal failure don't typically occur in these clients.
CN: Physiological integrity; CNS: Physiological adaptation; CL: Analysis

7. 1. Soft, smooth skin is a sign of adequate hydration. A sunken fontanel and no urine output in the first 24 hours of life are signs of poor hydration. In the case of no urine output, kidney dysfunction would also be a concern. Tachycardia, not bradycardia, may occur with dehydration.
CN: Physiological integrity; CNS: Physiological adaptation; CL: Analysis

CN: Client needs category   CNS: Client needs subcategory   CL: Cognitive level

8. When performing a neurologic assessment, which sign is considered a <u>normal</u> finding in a neonate?
1. Doll eyes
2. "Sunset" eyes
3. Positive Babinski's sign
4. Pupils that don't react to light

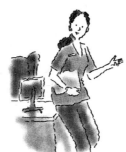

Question 8 asks what's *normal* versus what's *abnormal*. Be careful!

9. A nurse is caring for four clients on an antepartum unit. Which client would be carrying a viable conceptus at the earliest stage?
1. A client at 9 weeks' gestation
2. A client at 14 weeks' gestation
3. A client at 24 weeks' gestation
4. A client at 30 weeks' gestation

10. A client's mother asks the nurse why her newborn grandson is getting an injection of vitamin K. Which <u>best</u> explains why this drug is given to neonates?
1. Vitamin K assists with coagulation.
2. Vitamin K assists the gut to mature.
3. Vitamin K initiates the immunization process.
4. Vitamin K protects the brain from excess fluid production.

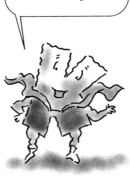

I'm very important to the well-being of a neonate. Do you know why?

11. A neonate is born to a woman infected with hepatitis B. Which treatment should be administered to this neonate?
1. Hepatitis B vaccine at birth and 1 month
2. Hepatitis B immune globulin at birth; no hepatitis B vaccine
3. Hepatitis B immune globulin within 48 hours of birth and hepatitis B vaccine at 1 month
4. Hepatitis B immune globulin within 12 hours of birth and hepatitis B vaccine at birth, 1 month, and 6 months

8. 3. A positive Babinski's sign is present in infants until approximately age 1. A positive Babinski's reflex is normal in neonates but abnormal in adults. Doll eyes is a neurologic response, but it's noted in adults. The appearance of "sunset" eyes, in which the sclera is visible above the iris, results from cranial nerve palsies and may indicate increased intracranial pressure. A neonate's pupils normally react to light as in an adult.
CN: Health promotion and maintenance; CNS: None; CL: Analysis

9. 3. At approximately 23 to 24 weeks' gestation, the lungs are developed enough to sometimes maintain extrauterine life. The lungs are the most immature system during the gestational period. Medical care for premature labor begins much earlier (aggressively at 21 weeks' gestation).
CN: Health promotion and maintenance; CNS: None; CL: Analysis

10. 1. Vitamin K, deficient in the neonate, is needed to activate clotting factors II, VII, IX, and X. In the event of trauma, the neonate would be at risk for excessive bleeding. Vitamin K doesn't assist the gut to mature, but the gut produces vitamin K after maturity is achieved. Vitamin K doesn't influence fluid production in the brain or the immunization process.
CN: Physiological integrity; CNS: Pharmacological and parenteral therapies; CL: Application

11. 4. Hepatitis B immune globulin should be given as soon as possible after birth but within 12 hours. Neonates should also receive hepatitis B vaccine at regularly scheduled intervals. This sequence of care has been determined as superior to the others provided.
CN: Health promotion and maintenance; CNS: None; CL: Analysis

12. When a neonate is delivered with meconium staining in the amniotic fluid, which sequence of events will most effectively <u>decrease</u> the risk of meconium aspiration?
   1. Deliver the thorax; then suction the nose.
   2. Clamp the umbilical cord; then suction the neonate's mouth.
   3. Deliver the head; then suction the mouth and then the nose.
   4. Deliver the thorax; then suction the nose and then the mouth.

13. Erythromycin ointment is administered to a neonate's eyes shortly after birth. The neonate's mother asks the nurse why this is done. The nurse tells the mother it is ordered to prevent which condition?
   1. Cataracts
   2. Diabetic retinopathy
   3. Ophthalmia neonatorum
   4. Strabismus

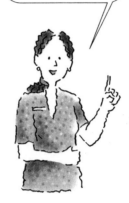

An ounce of prevention is worth a pound of cure!

14. A client with group AB blood whose husband has group O blood has just given birth. Which signs would indicate ABO blood incompatibility in the neonate?
   1. Negative Coombs' test
   2. Bleeding from the nose or ear
   3. Jaundice after the first 24 hours of life
   4. Jaundice within the first 24 hours of life

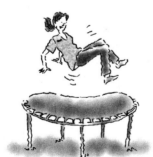

That's 15 questions down. Keep it up!

15. Which circumstance of delivery would predispose a neonate to respiratory distress syndrome (RDS)?
   1. Preterm birth
   2. Vaginal delivery
   3. First born of twins
   4. Postdate pregnancy

12. 3. To minimize the risk of aspiration of meconium after delivery, the neonate's mouth, then nose, should be suctioned after delivery of the head. This suctioning shouldn't be delayed until after delivery of the thorax because the neonate will take its first breath with meconium in its mouth.
CN: Physiological integrity; CN: Reduction of risk potential; CL: Analysis

13. 3. Eye prophylaxis is administered to the neonate immediately or soon after birth to prevent ophthalmia neonatorum. Cataracts are opacity of the lens of the eye associated with children with congenital rubella, galactosemia, and cortisone therapy. Diabetic retinopathy occurs in clients with diabetes when the retina bleeds into the vitreous, causing scarring, after which neovascularization occurs. Strabismus is neuromuscular incoordination of the eye alignment.
CN: Physiological integrity; CNS: Pharmacological and parenteral therapies; CL: Application

14. 4. The neonate with an ABO blood incompatibility with its mother will have jaundice within the first 24 hours of life. The neonate would have a positive Coombs' test result. Bleeding from the nose and ear should be investigated for possible causes but probably isn't related to ABO incompatibility. Jaundice after the first 24 hours of life is physiologic jaundice.
CN: Physiological integrity; CNS: Reduction of risk potential; CL: Analysis

15. 1. Preterm birth is the single most important risk factor for developing RDS. The second born of twins and neonates born by cesarean delivery are also at increased risk for RDS. Surfactant deficiency, which commonly results in RDS, isn't a problem for postdate neonates.
CN: Physiological integrity; CNS: Physiological adaptation; CL: Analysis

CN: Client needs category   CNS: Client needs subcategory   CL: Cognitive level

16. Two days after circumcision, a nurse notes a yellow-white exudate around the head of the neonate's penis. What would be the <u>most</u> appropriate nursing intervention?
1. Leave the area alone.
2. Report the findings to the physician.
3. Take the neonate's temperature.
4. Remove the exudate with a warm washcloth.

17. A client has just given birth at 42 weeks' gestation. When assessing the neonate, which physical finding is expected?
1. A sleepy, lethargic baby
2. Lanugo covering the body
3. Desquamation of the epidermis
4. Vernix caseosa covering the body

18. A client delivers a small-for-gestation neonate. Which complication is this neonate most at risk for developing?
1. Anemia probably due to chronic fetal hypoxia
2. Hyperthermia due to decreased glycogen stores
3. Hyperglycemia due to decreased glycogen stores
4. Polycythemia probably due to chronic fetal hypoxia

19. Which finding might be seen in a neonate suspected of having an infection?
1. Flushed cheeks
2. Increased temperature
3. Decreased temperature
4. Increased activity level

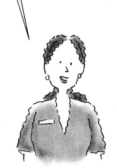

The color of an exudate helps determine its cause.

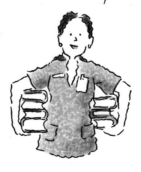

The test-taking expertise you're gaining from answering these questions will be well worth the effort you're putting in. Keep at it!

16. 1. The yellow-white exudate is part of the granulation process and a normal finding for a healing penis after circumcision. Therefore, notifying the physician isn't necessary. There's no indication of an infection that would necessitate taking the neonate's temperature. The exudate shouldn't be removed.
CN: Health promotion and maintenance; CNS: None; CL: Analysis

17. 3. Postdate fetuses lose the vernix caseosa, and the epidermis may become desquamated. These neonates are usually very alert. Lanugo is missing in the postdate neonate.
CN: Health promotion and maintenance; CNS: None; CL: Application

18. 4. The small-for-gestation neonate is at risk for developing polycythemia (not anemia) because of a state of anoxia during intrauterine life. The neonates are also at increased risk for developing hypoglycemia and hypothermia due to decreased glycogen stores.
CN: Health promotion and maintenance; CNS: None; CL: Analysis

19. 3. Temperature instability, especially when it results in a low temperature in the neonate, may be a sign of infection. The neonate's color commonly changes with an infection process but generally becomes ashen or mottled. The neonate with an infection will usually show a decrease in activity level or lethargy.
CN: Physiological integrity; CNS: Physiological adaptation; CL: Analysis

20. A neonate has just been delivered without incident. Which symptom would indicate successful adaptation to extrauterine life?
1. Nasal flaring
2. Light audible grunting
3. Respiratory rate 40 to 60 breaths/minute
4. Apgar score of 5

21. After reviewing the client's maternal history of magnesium sulfate during labor, which condition should the nurse anticipate as a potential problem in the neonate?
1. Hypoglycemia
2. Jitteriness
3. Respiratory depression
4. Tachycardia

22. Which intervention is helpful for the neonate experiencing drug withdrawal?
1. Place the isolette in a quiet area of the nursery.
2. Withhold all medication to improve the liver's metabolization of drugs.
3. Dress the neonate in loose clothing so he won't feel restricted.
4. Place the isolette near the nurses' station for frequent contact with health care workers.

23. A client with gestational diabetes delivers a neonate. Because of the client's gestational diabetes, which complication is the neonate at risk for following birth?
1. Atelectasis
2. Microcephaly
3. Pneumothorax
4. Macrosomia

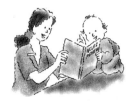

It's time to adapt to the "outside of the womb" world.

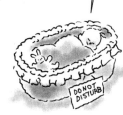

I need special interventions… whatever that means.

20. 3. A respiratory rate 40 to 60 breaths/minute is normal for a neonate during the transitional period. Nasal flaring and audible grunting are signs of respiratory distress. An Apgar score of 5 or less indicates a need for resuscitative efforts.
CN: Health maintenance and promotion; CNS: None; CL: Analysis

21. 3. Magnesium sulfate crosses the placenta, and adverse neonatal effects are respiratory depression, hypotonia, and bradycardia. The serum blood sugar isn't affected by magnesium sulfate. The neonate would be floppy, not jittery.
CN: Physiological integrity; CNS: Pharmacological and parenteral therapies; CL: Analysis

22. 1. Neonates experiencing drug withdrawal commonly have sleep disturbance. The neonate should be moved to a quiet area of the nursery to minimize environmental stimuli. Medications, such as phenobarbital and paregoric, should be given as needed. The neonate should be swaddled to prevent him from flailing and stimulating himself.
CN: Psychosocial integrity; CNS: None; CL: Analysis

23. 4. Neonates of mothers with diabetes are at increased risk for macrosomia (excessive fetal growth) as a result of the combination of the increased supply of maternal glucose and an increase in fetal insulin. Along with macrosomia, neonates of diabetic mothers are at risk for respiratory distress syndrome, hypoglycemia, hypocalcemia, hyperbilirubinemia, and congenital anomalies. They aren't at greater risk for atelectasis or pneumothorax. Microcephaly is usually the result of cytomegalovirus or rubella virus infection.
CN: Health promotion and maintenance; CNS: None; CL: Analysis

CN: Client needs category   CNS: Client needs subcategory   CL: Cognitive level

24. A neonate is diagnosed with hemorrhagic disease. Which medication should have been given to the neonate as a <u>preventive</u> measure?
1. Vitamin K
2. Heparin
3. Iron
4. Warfarin

25. Which places a neonate at an increased risk for losing heat during the transition period?
1. Placing a cap on the neonate's head immediately after delivery
2. Preheating the radiant warmer prior to delivery
3. Placing the thermometer on the shelf of the radiant warmer
4. Wrapping the neonate in the same blankets used for drying

26. A nursery nurse wraps a neonate in a blanket and keeps the nursery temperature warm. Which type of heat loss is she trying to prevent in the neonate?
1. Conduction
2. Convection
3. Evaporation
4. Radiation

27. A nurse is explaining physiologic hyperbilirubinemia to the parents of a neonate. Which statement made by one of the parents would demonstrate a correct understanding of the concept?
1. "The neonate usually also has a medical problem."
2. "In term neonates, it usually appears after 24 hours."
3. "It's caused by elevated conjugated bilirubin levels."
4. "It's usually progressive from the neonate's feet to his head."

Which measure is preventive, rather than curative or restorative?

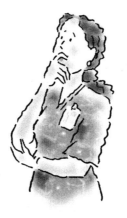

Be careful with this prefix. Hyper is almost identical to hypo, but its meaning, of course, is vastly different.

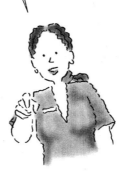

24. 1. Neonates have coagulation deficiencies because of a lack of organisms that help produce vitamin K in the intestines, which helps the liver synthesize clotting factors II, VII, IX, and X. Heparin and warfarin are given as anticoagulant therapy, not to prevent hemorrhagic disease in the neonate. Iron is stored in the fetal liver; hemoglobin binds to iron and carries oxygen.
CN: Health promotion and maintenance; CNS: None; CL: Application

25. 4. Wrapping the infant in the previously used wet blankets causes continued heat loss by evaporation. Placing a cap on the neonate's head immediately after delivery, preheating the radiant warmer, and placing objects outside of the crib helps prevent heat loss.
CN: Health promotion and maintenance; CNS: None; CL: Application

26. 2. Convection heat loss is the flow of heat from the body surface to cooler air. Conduction is the loss of heat from the body surface to cooler surfaces in direct contact. Evaporation is the loss of heat that occurs when a liquid is converted to a vapor. Radiation is the loss of heat from the body surface to cooler solid surfaces not in direct contact but in relative proximity.
CN: Health promotion and maintenance; CNS: None; CL: Application

27. 2. Physiologic jaundice in term neonates first appears after 24 hours. Neonates are otherwise healthy and have no medical problems. Hyperbilirubinemia is caused almost exclusively from unconjugated bilirubin. Jaundice usually appears in a cephalocaudal progression from head to feet.
CN: Physiological integrity; CNS: Reduction of risk potential; CL: Analysis

28. A neonate has been diagnosed with caput succedaneum. Which information should the nurse include while teaching the mother about caput succedaneum?
1. It usually resolves in 3 to 6 weeks.
2. It doesn't cross the cranial suture line.
3. It's a collection of blood between the skull and periosteum.
4. It involves swelling of the tissue over the presenting part of the fetal head.

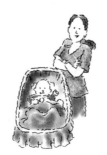

When you're teaching a new mom, it helps to know what to expect at each stage in a neonate's development!

29. A postpartum client expresses concern about the look of her baby's first stool, which she describes as "dark and slimy." Which is the best statement for the nurse to make for patient education?
1. "These types of stools occur when the baby is dehydrated in utero."
2. "The physician will be notified about this abnormal occurrence when he examines the infant."
3. "This bowel movement is called meconium and is considered normal."
4. "The type of first stool for your baby is determined by your diet during pregnancy."

30. A 3-day-old neonate needs phototherapy for hyperbilirubinemia. Nursery care of a neonate receiving phototherapy should include which nursing intervention?
1. Tube feedings
2. Feeding the neonate under phototherapy lights
3. Mask over the eyes to prevent retinal damage
4. Temperature monitored every 6 hours during phototherapy

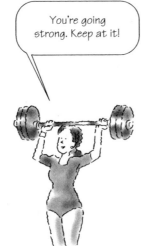

You're going strong. Keep at it!

31. A nurse is caring for four neonates. Which neonate is most likely to develop hyperbilirubinemia?
1. Neonate of an African-American mother
2. Neonate of an Rh-positive mother
3. Neonate with ABO incompatibility
4. Neonate with Apgar scores 9 and 10 at 1 and 5 minutes

28. 4. Caput succedaneum is the swelling of tissue over the presenting part of the fetal scalp due to sustained pressure. This boggy edematous swelling is present at birth, crosses the suture line, and most commonly occurs in the occipital area. A cephalhematoma is a collection of blood between the skull and periosteum that doesn't cross cranial suture lines and resolves in 3 to 6 weeks. Caput succedaneum resolves within 3 to 4 days.
CN: Physiological integrity; CNS: Physiological adaptation; CL: Application

29. 3. Meconium collects in the GI tract during gestation and is initially sterile. Meconium is greenish black because of occult blood and is viscous. Dehydration in utero does not occur. Physician notification is not necessary, as this is a normal occurrence for the first bowel movement. The stool of a neonate is not affected by the mother's antenatal diet.
CN: Health promotion and maintenance; CNS: None; CL: Analysis

30. 3. The neonate's eyes and genitalia must be covered with eye patches to prevent damage. The neonate can be removed from the lights and held for feeding. The neonate's temperature should be monitored at least every 2 to 4 hours because of the risk of hyperthermia with phototherapy.
CN: Physiological integrity; CNS: Physiological adaptation; CL: Analysis

31. 3. The mother's blood type, which is different from the neonate's, has an impact on the neonate's bilirubin level because of the antigen-antibody reaction. African-American neonates tend to have lower mean levels of bilirubin. Chinese, Japanese, Korean, and Greek neonates tend to have higher incidences of hyperbilirubinemia. Neonates of Rh-negative, not Rh-positive, mothers tend to have hyperbilirubinemia. Low Apgar scores may indicate a risk of hyperbilirubinemia.
CN: Physiological integrity; CNS: Physiological adaptation; CL: Analysis

CN: Client needs category   CNS: Client needs subcategory   CL: Cognitive level

32. A neonate has developed a major infection. Which gram-positive bacteria most likely contributed to this problem?
1. *Escherichia coli*
2. Group B streptococci
3. *Klebsiella* species
4. *Pseudomonas aeruginosa*

33. A neonate develops sepsis 18 hours after birth. Which organism most likely contributed to this problem?
1. *Candida albicans*
2. *Chlamydia trachomatis*
3. *Escherichia coli*
4. Group B beta-hemolytic streptococci

34. A nurse administers erythromycin ointment to a neonate's eyes to:
1. eliminate the incidence of viral infections.
2. prevent chlamydia infections.
3. prevent syphilis infection of the eyes.
4. reduce the incidence of group B streptococcal conjunctivitis.

35. When attempting to interact with a neonate experiencing drug withdrawal, which behavior would indicate that the neonate is willing to interact?
1. Gaze aversion
2. Hiccups
3. Quiet, alert state
4. Yawning

36. When teaching umbilical cord care to a new mother, a nurse would include which information?
1. Apply peroxide to the cord with each diaper change.
2. Cover the cord with petroleum jelly after bathing.
3. Use alcohol on the cord; keep it dry and open to air.
4. Wash the cord with soap and water each day during a tub bath.

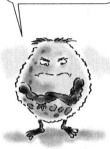

I'm responsible and proud of it!

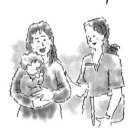

The stump of the umbilical cord will fall off later.

32. 2. Group B streptococci are gram-positive cocci that the neonate is exposed to if these bacteria are colonized in the vaginal tract. *E. coli, Klebsiella,* and *P. aeruginosa* species are gram-negative rods that produce 78% to 85% of the bacterial infection in neonates.
CN: Physiological integrity; CNS: Physiological adaptation; CL: Analysis

33. 4. Transmission of group B beta-hemolytic streptococci to the fetus results in respiratory distress that can rapidly lead to septic shock. *E. coli* is the second most common cause. Candidiasis may be acquired from the birth canal and causes infection later than 24 hours. *C. trachomatis* infection causes neonatal conjunctivitis and pneumonia.
CN: Physiological integrity; CNS: Physiological adaptation; CL: Analysis

34. 2. Both chlamydia and gonorrhea are common causes of neonatal conjunctival infections, and erythromycin effectively treats these infections. Viral infections aren't treated with antibiotics, and syphilis and group B streptococcal infections are treated with other antibiotics.
CN: Physiological integrity; CNS: Pharmacological and parenteral therapies; CL: Analysis

35. 3. When caring for a neonate experiencing drug withdrawal, the nurse needs to be alert for distress signals from the neonate. Stimuli should be introduced one at a time when the neonate is in a quiet alert state. Gaze aversion, yawning, sneezing, hiccups, and body arching are distress signals that the neonate can't handle stimuli at that time.
CN: Psychosocial integrity; CNS: None; CL: Analysis

36. 3. Using alcohol on the cord and keeping it dry and open to air helps reduce infection and hastens drying. Peroxide could be painful and isn't recommended. Petroleum jelly prevents the cord from drying and encourages infection. Infants aren't given tub baths but are sponged off until the cord falls off.
CN: Health promotion and maintenance; CNS: None CL: Application

37. When caring for an infant of a mother with diabetes, which physiological finding is <u>most</u> indicative of a hypoglycemic episode?
1. Hyperalert state
2. Jitteriness
3. Excessive crying
4. Serum glucose level of 60 mg/dl

38. A mother of a term neonate asks what the thick, white, cheesy coating is on his skin. Which statement correctly describes the function of this coating for the neonate?
1. It helps keep the neonate warm after birth.
2. It prevents neonatal dehydration after birth.
3. It serves as a protective coating in utero.
4. It decreases the development of birth marks.

39. Which drug is <u>routinely</u> given to the neonate within 1 hour of birth?
1. Erythromycin ophthalmic ointment
2. Gentamicin
3. Nystatin
4. Vitamin A

40. Which condition or treatment <u>best</u> ensures lung maturity in a neonate?
1. Meconium in the amniotic fluid
2. Glucocorticoid treatment just before delivery
3. Lecithin to sphingomyelin ratio more than 2:1
4. Absence of phosphatidylglycerol in amniotic fluid

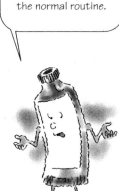

What can I say? I'm just part of the normal routine.

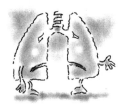

Why do they think I'm immature?

37. 2. Hypoglycemia in a neonate is expressed as jitteriness, lethargy, diaphoresis, and a serum glucose level below 40 mg/dl. A hyperalert state in a neonate is more suggestive of neurologic irritability and has no correlation to blood glucose levels. Excessive crying isn't found in hypoglycemia. A serum glucose level of 60 mg/dl is a normal level.
CN: Physiological integrity; CNS: Physiological adaptation; CL: Analysis

38. 3. Vernix caseosa is a white, cheesy material present on the neonate's skin at birth. The purpose of the vernix caseosa is to protect the fetus in utero. It does not prevent dehydration or keep the neonate warm after birth. There is no association between vernix caseosa and birthmarks.
CN: Health promotion and maintenance; CNS: None; CL: Analysis

39. 1. Erythromycin ophthalmic ointment is given for prophylactic treatment of ophthalmic neonatorum. Gentamicin is an antibiotic used in the treatment of an infection of the neonate. Nystatin is used for treatment of neonate thrush. Vitamin K, not vitamin A, is given.
CN: Physiological integrity; CNS: Pharmacological and parenteral therapies; CL: Analysis

40. 3. Lecithin and sphingomyelin are phospholipids that help compose surfactant in the lungs; lecithin peaks at 36 weeks, and sphingomyelin concentrations remain stable. Meconium is released because of fetal stress before delivery, but it's chronic fetal stress that matures lungs. Glucocorticoids must be given at least 48 hours before delivery. The presence of phosphatidylglycerol indicates lung maturity.
CN: Physiological integrity; CNS: Physiological adaptation; CL: Analysis

CN: Client needs category   CNS: Client needs subcategory   CL: Cognitive level

41. Which assessment finding would place the neonate at the least risk for developing respiratory distress syndrome (RDS)?
1. Second born of twins
2. Neonate born at 34 weeks
3. Neonate of a diabetic mother
4. Chronic maternal hypertension

42. A nurse is performing an assessment on a neonate. Which finding is considered common in the healthy neonate?
1. Simian crease
2. Conjunctival hemorrhages
3. Cystic hygroma
4. Bulging fontanelle

43. When performing nursing care for a neonate after a birth, which intervention has the highest nursing priority?
1. Obtain a Dextrostix.
2. Give the initial bath.
3. Give the vitamin K injection.
4. Cover the neonate's wet head with a cap.

44. When assessing a neonate's skin, the nurse observes small, white papules surrounded by erythematous dermatitis. Which most accurately describes this condition?
1. Cutis marmorata
2. Epstein's pearls
3. Erythema toxicum
4. Mongolian spots

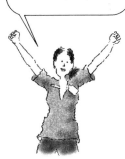

Congratulations! You're halfway through this chapter.

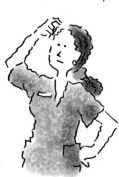

Which one of these actions is a priority right after birth?

41. 4. Chronic maternal hypertension is an unlikely factor because chronic fetal stress tends to increase lung maturity. The second born of twins may be prone to greater risk of asphyxia leading to RDS. Premature neonates younger than 36 weeks are associated with RDS. Even with a mature lecithin to sphingomyelin ratio, neonates of mothers with diabetes may still develop respiratory distress.
CN: Physiological integrity; CNS: Physiological adaptation; CL: Analysis

42. 2. Conjunctival hemorrhages are commonly seen in neonates secondary to the cranial pressure applied during the birth process. Simian creases are present in 40% of the neonates with trisomy 21. Cystic hygroma is a neck mass that can affect the airway. Bulging fontanelles are a sign of intracranial pressure.
CN: Health promotion and maintenance; CNS: None; CL: Analysis

43. 3. The American Academy of Pediatrics recommends that vitamin K be given in the delivery room within 1 hour of birth. Dextrostix, appropriate for neonates with risk factors, are obtained at 30 minutes to 1 hour of age. Initial baths aren't given until the neonate's temperature is stable. The head shouldn't be covered until the hair is dried under a radiant warmer.
CN: Safe, effective care environment; CNS: Management of care; CL: Analysis

44. 3. Erythema toxicum has lesions that come and go on the face, trunk, and limbs. They're small, white or yellow papules or vesicles with erythematous dermatitis and resemble flea bites. Cutis marmorata is bluish mottling of the skin. Epstein's pearls, found in the mouth, are similar to facial milia. Mongolian spots are large macules or patches that are gray or blue green.
CN: Health promotion and maintenance; CNS: None; CL: Application

45. Which nursing consideration is <u>most important</u> when giving a neonate his initial bath?
1. Give a tub bath.
2. Use water and mild soap.
3. Give it right after delivery.
4. Use hexachlorophene soap.

46. The nurse is teaching the parents of a neonate about the Centers for Disease Control and Prevention (CDC) recommendations for hepatitis B vaccine. Which statement would be the most accurate concerning these recommendations?
1. "It should be given to all neonates."
2. "It should be given to neonates exposed to hepatitis B only."
3. "It should be given to neonates showing symptoms of hepatitis B."
4. "It should be given to neonates whose mothers have human immunodeficiency virus."

47. A male neonate has just been circumcised. Which nursing intervention is part of the initial care of a circumcised neonate?
1. Apply alcohol to the site.
2. Change the diaper as needed.
3. Keep the neonate in the supine position.
4. Apply petroleum gauze to the site for 24 hours.

48. When performing an assessment on a neonate, which assessment finding is <u>most suggestive</u> of hypothermia?
1. Bradycardia
2. Hyperglycemia
3. Metabolic alkalosis
4. Shivering

49. Which nursing intervention helps <u>prevent</u> evaporative heat loss in the neonate immediately after birth?
1. Administering warm oxygen
2. Controlling the drafts in the room
3. Immediately drying the neonate
4. Placing the neonate on a warm, dry towel

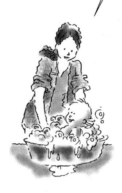

What's most important for baby's first bath?

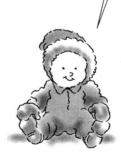

I'm sure to stay warm now.

45. 2. Use only water and mild soap on a neonate to prevent drying out the skin. The initial bath is given when the neonate's temperature is stable. Tub baths are delayed until the umbilical cord falls off. Hexachlorophene soaps should be avoided; they're neurotoxic and may be absorbed through a neonate's skin.
CN: Health promotion and maintenance; CNS: None; CL: Application

46. 1. The CDC recommends hepatitis B vaccine be given to all neonates, including those born to hepatitis B surface antigen–negative mothers, before hospital discharge.
CN: Health promotion and maintenance; CNS: None; CL: Application

47. 4. Petroleum gauze is applied to the site for the first 24 hours to prevent the skin edges from sticking to the diaper. Alcohol is contraindicated for circumcision care. Diapers are changed more frequently to inspect the site. Neonates are initially kept in the prone position.
CN: Health promotion and maintenance; CNS: None; CL: Application

48. 1. Hypothermic neonates become bradycardic proportional to the degree of core temperature. Hypoglycemia is seen in hypothermic neonates. Metabolic acidosis, not alkalosis, is seen as a result of slowed respirations. Neonates use nonshivering thermogenesis.
CN: Health promotion and maintenance; CNS: None; CL: Analysis

49. 3. Immediately drying the neonate decreases evaporative heat loss from his moist body from birth. Controlling the drafts in the room and administering warmed oxygen help reduce convective loss. Placing the neonate on a warm, dry towel decreases conductive losses.
CN: Health promotion and maintenance; CNS: None; CL: Analysis

CN: Client needs category   CNS: Client needs subcategory   CL: Cognitive level

50. A nurse is performing an assessment on a neonate. Which assessment finding would indicate a metabolic response to cold stress?
1. Arrhythmias
2. Hypoglycemia
3. Increase in liver function
4. Increase in blood pressure

51. Which would be the highest priority in regulating the temperature of a neonate?
1. Supply extra heat sources to the neonate.
2. Keep the ambient room temperature less than 100° F (37.8°C).
3. Minimize the energy needed for the neonate to produce heat.
4. Block radiant, convective, conductive, and evaporative losses.

52. Which neonate would be most at risk for a problem with thermoregulation?
1. A term neonate born to a diabetic mother.
2. A preterm neonate born at 36 weeks' gestation.
3. A preterm neonate born at 39 weeks' gestation.
4. A term neonate with signs of jaundice at 36 hours of age.

53. Which clinical finding is most suggestive of physiologic hyperbilirubinemia in a neonate?
1. Clinical jaundice before 36 hours of age
2. Clinical jaundice lasting beyond 14 days
3. Bilirubin levels of 12 mg/dl by 3 days of life
4. Serum bilirubin level increasing by more than 5 mg/dl/day

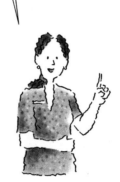

The word *highest* is a clue to the answer!

Sometimes timing is everything!

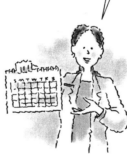

50. 2. Hypoglycemia occurs as the consumption of glucose increases with the increase in metabolic rate. Arrhythmias and increases in blood pressure occur because of cardiorespiratory manifestations. Liver function declines in cold stress.
CN: Health promotion and maintenance; CNS: None; CL: Analysis

51. 4. Prevention of heat loss is always the first goal in thermoregulation to avoid hypothermia. The second goal is to minimize the energy necessary for neonates to produce heat. Adding extra heat sources is a means of correcting hypothermia. The ambient room temperature should be kept at approximately 100°F.
CN: Safe, effective care environment; CNS: Management of care; CL: Application

52. 2. Preterm neonates are not able to thermoregulate due to the lack of brown fat. The more premature the infant, the more immature the thermoregulation system. Infants born to diabetic mothers and those with jaundice are not more at risk for problems with thermoregulation than a premature infant.
CN: Physiological integrity; CNS: Reduction of risk potential; CL: Analysis

53. 3. Increased bilirubin levels in the liver usually cause bilirubin levels of 12 mg/dl by the 3rd day of life. This is from the impaired conjugation and excretion of bilirubin and difficulty clearing bilirubin from plasma. The other answers suggest pathologic jaundice.
CN: Physiological integrity; CNS: Reduction of risk potential; CL: Analysis

54. A nurse is caring for a full-term neonate who's receiving phototherapy for hyperbilirubinemia. She should notify the physician immediately if which finding is noted?
1. Maculopapular rash
2. Absent Moro reflex
3. Greenish stools
4. Bronze-colored skin

55. A neonate undergoing phototherapy treatment needs to be monitored for which adverse effect?
1. Hyperglycemia
2. Increased insensible water loss
3. Severe decrease in platelet count
4. Increased GI transit time

56. Which assessment finding might be seen in a neonate suspected of having early breast-milk jaundice?
1. History of being a poor feeder
2. Decreased bilirubin level around day 3 of life
3. Clinical jaundice evident after 24 hours
4. Interruption of breast-feeding resulting in decreased bilirubin levels between 24 and 72 hours

57. Which sign is the earliest indication of respiratory distress syndrome (RDS) in a neonate?
1. Bilateral crackles
2. Pale gray color
3. Tachypnea more than 60 breaths/minute
4. Poor capillary filling time (3 to 4 seconds)

58. A nurse is caring for a neonate with respiratory problems. Which condition is most likely to be caused by fluid remaining in the lungs of the neonate after delivery?
1. Choanal atresia
2. Meconium aspiration
3. Pulmonary hemorrhage
4. Transient tachypnea of a newborn

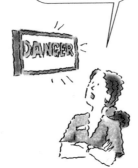

The signs are pointing to a dangerous situation.

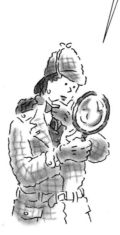

It's important to recognize the earliest clue.

54. 2. An absent Moro reflex, lethargy, and seizures are symptoms of bilirubin encephalopathy which can be life-threatening. A maculopapular rash, greenish stools, and bronze-colored skin are minor side effects of phototherapy that should be monitored but don't require immediate intervention.
CN: Physiological integrity; CNS: Physiological adaptation; CL: Analysis

55. 2. Increased insensible water loss is due to absorbed photon energy from the lights. Hyperglycemia isn't a characteristic effect of phototherapy treatment. There may be a mild decrease in platelet count. GI transit time may decrease with use of phototherapy.
CN: Health promotion and maintenance; CNS: None; CL: Analysis

56. 4. The exact cause of early breast-milk jaundice is unknown. If bilirubin levels don't decrease after 3 days, human milk is eliminated as a cause. These babies are typically good eaters with good weight gain. Bilirubin levels increase, rather than decrease, at day 3. Jaundice in the first 24 hours of life is characteristic of hemolytic disease.
CN: Health promotion and maintenance; CNS: None; CL: Analysis

57. 3. Tachypnea and expiratory grunting occur early in RDS to help improve oxygenation. Crackles occur as the respiratory distress progressively worsens. A pale gray skin color obscures earlier cyanosis as respiratory distress symptoms persist and worsen. Poor capillary filling time, a later manifestation, occurs if signs and symptoms aren't treated.
CN: Health promotion and maintenance; CNS: None; CL: Analysis

58. 4. Transient tachypnea of a newborn is caused by a delay in removing excessive amounts of lung fluid. Choanal atresia is caused by a protrusion of bone or membrane into nasal passages, causing blockage or narrowing. Meconium aspiration is meconium aspirated into the lungs during birth. Pulmonary hemorrhage is bleeding into the alveoli.
CN: Physiological integrity; CNS: Physiological adaptation; CL: Analysis

CN: Client needs category   CNS: Client needs subcategory   CL: Cognitive level

59. A neonate is admitted to the neonatal intensive care unit with persistent pulmonary hypertension. Which pulmonary vasodilator is the drug of choice for this disorder?
1. Dobutamine
2. Isoproterenol (Isuprel)
3. Prostaglandin E_2
4. Inhaled nitric oxide

60. Which neonatal respiratory disorder is usually mild and runs a self-limited course?
1. Pneumonia
2. Meconium aspiration syndrome
3. Transient tachypnea of newborn
4. Persistent pulmonary hypertension

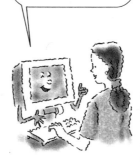

You've reached question 60. Outstanding!

61. Which procedure should be <u>avoided</u> in a neonate born with diaphragmatic hernia?
1. Chest X-ray
2. Mask ventilation
3. Placement of orogastric tube
4. Immediate endotracheal intubation

62. A nurse is preparing to administer Survanta (Beractant) to a preterm infant. The order is for 4 ml/kg. The neonate weighs 2000 grams. How many total ml will be used for one dose? Record your answer as a whole number:
_____ml

63. A nurse is caring for a neonate with fetal alcohol syndrome (FAS). Which craniofacial change is most indicative of FAS?
1. Macrocephaly
2. Microophthalmia
3. Wide palpebral fissures
4. Well-developed philtrum

59. 4. Inhaled nitric oxide is a potent selective pulmonary vasodilator. Dobutamine is a vasopressor, not a vasodilator. Isoproterenol dilates pulmonary arteries but doesn't decrease pulmonary vascular resistance. Prostaglandin E_2 is an oxytocic substance used to induce abortion and doesn't affect pulmonary vasodilation.
CN: Physiological integrity; CNS: Pharmacological and parenteral therapies; CL: Analysis

60. 3. Transient tachypnea has an invariably favorable outcome after several hours to several days. The outcome of pneumonia depends on the causative agent involved and may have complications. Meconium aspiration, depending on severity, may have long-term adverse effects. In persistent pulmonary hypertension, the mortality rate is more than 50%.
CN: Physiological integrity; CNS: Physiological adaptation; CL: Analysis

61. 2. Mask ventilation should be avoided to prevent air from being introduced into the GI tract by this technique. An emergency chest X-ray will help in diagnosing this defect. An orogastric tube is needed to decompress the bowel and stomach within the chest. Intubation is needed to ventilate the neonate because of the defect.
CN: Physiological integrity; CNS: Physiological adaptation; CL: Application

62. 8. The answer is 8 ml.
First, convert the weight from grams to kilograms using the conversion:
1000 gm = 1 kg
1000 gm/1 kg = 2000 gm/x kg
X = 2 kg
Then, determine how many ml are needed by using the following formula:
4 ml × 2 kg = 8 ml total dose.
CN: Physiological integrity; CNS: Pharmacological and parenteral therapies; CL: Application

63. 2. Distinctive facial dysmorphology of children with FAS most commonly involves the eyes (microophthalmia). Microcephaly is generally seen, as are short palpebral fissures and a poorly developed philtrum.
CN: Physiological integrity; CNS: Physiological adaptation; CL: Analysis

64. A 36-week neonate born weighing 1,800 g has microcephaly and microophthalmia. Based on these findings, which risk factor might be <u>expected</u> in the maternal history?
1. Use of alcohol
2. Use of marijuana
3. Gestational diabetes
4. Positive group B streptococci

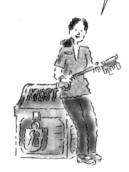

The mother's history may be the key to the neonate's current condition.

65. Which condition requires intervention when displayed by a neonate born to a mother with a history of chronic alcohol abuse?
1. Hypoactivity
2. High birth weight
3. Poor wake and sleep patterns
4. High threshold of stimulation

66. A neonate is admitted to rule out a diagnosis of cystic fibrosis. Which GI disorder <u>most likely</u> indicates this diagnosis?
1. Duodenal obstruction
2. Jejunal atresia
3. Malrotation
4. Meconium ileus

67. During discharge instructions, which statement by the nurse would be the most correct for the safety of the neonate? Select all that apply:
1. "Heavy blankets or stuffed animals can be placed in the crib."
2. "The car seat used should be a front-facing model."
3. "Never leave your infant alone in the tub."
4. "Verify that you babysitter knows CPR."
5. "The car seat used should be a rear-facing model."

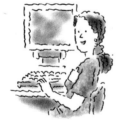

Keep reading each question carefully and you'll do well.

68. A neonate has an imperforate anus, tracheoesophageal fistula, and a single umbilical artery. A nurse suspects that the neonate might have which congenital disorder?
1. Beckwith-Wiedemann syndrome
2. Trisomy 13
3. Turner's syndrome
4. VATER association

64. 1. The most common sign of the effects of alcohol on fetal development is retarded growth in weight, length, and head circumference. Intrauterine growth retardation isn't characteristic of marijuana use. Gestational diabetes usually produces large-for-gestational-age neonates. Positive group B streptococcus isn't a relevant risk factor.
CN: Health promotion and maintenance; CNS: None; CL: Analysis

65. 3. Altered sleep patterns are caused by disturbances in the central nervous system from alcohol exposure in utero. Hyperactivity is a characteristic deficit generally associated with fetal alcohol syndrome (FAS). Low birth weight is a physical defect seen in neonates with FAS. Neonates with FAS generally have a low threshold for stimulation.
CN: Physiological integrity; CNS: Physiological adaptation; CL: Application

66. 4. Meconium ileus is a luminal obstruction of the distal small intestine by abnormal meconium seen in neonates with cystic fibrosis. Duodenal obstruction, jejunal atresia, and malrotation aren't characteristic findings in neonates with cystic fibrosis.
CN: Physiological integrity; CNS: Physiological adaptation; CL: Analysis

67. 3, 4, 5. Infants should never be left alone in the tub, as they can easily drown. All caretakers should be trained in CPR. Car seats should be rear-facing models, not front-facing models, until the infant weights 20 pounds and/or is one-year-old. Heavy blankets or stuffed animals in the crib increase the risk of sudden infant death syndrome (SIDS).
CN: Health promotion and maintenance; CNS: None; CL: Application

68. 4. VATER association clinically presents with three or more defects, including the three mentioned. These defects aren't associated with Beckwith-Wiedemann syndrome. Trisomy 13 and Turner's syndrome are chromosomal aberrations that aren't typically seen with the other defects.
CN: Physiological integrity; CNS: Physiological adaptation; CL: Analysis

69. An initial assessment of a female neonate shows pink-streaked vaginal discharge. This data indicates which condition?
1. Cystitis
2. Birth trauma
3. Neonatal candidiasis
4. Withdrawal of maternal hormones

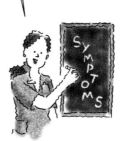

Question 70 asks about early signs of tracheoesophageal atresia.

70. When assessing for congenital anomalies in a neonate, which symptom is seen <u>first</u> with tracheoesophageal atresia?
1. Torticollis
2. Nasal stuffiness
3. Oligohydramnios
4. Excessive oral secretions

71. A new mother states to the nurse, "My baby spits up after every feeding." Which intervention would be appropriate to teach the mother initially for this problem?
1. Feed the baby every hour.
2. Change the infant to a soy formula.
3. Lay the infant on its stomach after every feeding.
4. Burp the infant more frequently during each feeding.

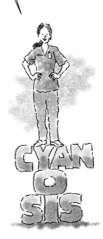

You need to stay on top of central cyanosis in a neonate.

72. Maintaining thermoregulation in the neonate is an important nursing intervention because cold stress in the neonate can lead to which condition?
1. Anemia
2. Hyperglycemia
3. Metabolic alkalosis
4. Increased oxygen consumption

73. Which initial nursing intervention best addresses the needs of a term neonate with adequate respiratory and heart rates but who has central cyanosis?
1. Provide tactile stimulation.
2. Give supplemental free-flow oxygen.
3. Assist ventilation with a bag and mask.
4. Intubate and suction the lower airway.

69. 4. Withdrawal of maternal estrogen can produce pseudomenstruation. Cystitis or a urinary tract infection in a neonate would show generalized signs of sepsis. Birth trauma may cause surface abrasions but not vaginal discharge. Neonates with candidal infections usually have oral lesions (thrush) or monilial diaper rash.
CN: Health promotion and maintenance; CNS: None; CL: Application

70. 4. Accumulated secretions are copious in neonates with this disorder because the neonate can't swallow. Torticollis would be present only if there was a defect of muscle or bone. Nasal stuffiness is very common in neonates and doesn't indicate esophageal abnormalities. Atresia will produce polyhydramnios because the fetus can't swallow the amniotic fluid.
CN: Physiological integrity; CNS: Physiological adaptation; CL: Analysis

71. 4. Frequent burping decreases the amount of air the infant has in it stomach. Laying an infant on its back or side after feeding is preferred. Formula may have to be changed if it is determined that the spitting is related to milk intolerance, but this is not the initial reaction. Infants should be fed every 2–4 hours.
CN: Health promotion and maintenance; CNS: None; CL: Analysis

72. 4. The neonate's metabolic rate increases as a result of cold stress, which leads to an increased oxygen requirement. Cold stress doesn't increase erythrocyte destruction. Cold stress leads to anaerobic glycolysis, which results in metabolic acidosis. The increased metabolic rate leads to the use of glycogen stores and produces hypoglycemia.
CN: Physiological integrity; CNS: Reduction of risk potential; CL: Analysis

73. 2. Room air is currently insufficient, seen by the central cyanosis. Tactile stimulation is needed only if the neonate is apneic or gasping. Bag and mask ventilation is indicated only if the heart rate is less than 100 beats/minute. Intubation is indicated only in special circumstances, such as prematurity or a diaphragmatic hernia.
CN: Health promotion and maintenance; CNS: None; CL: Application

74. A woman delivers a 3,250-g neonate at 42 weeks' gestation. Which physical finding is <u>expected</u> during an examination of this neonate?

1. Abundant lanugo
2. Absence of sole creases
3. Breast bud of 1 to 2 mm in diameter
4. Leathery, cracked, and wrinkled skin

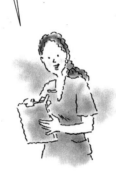

Question 74 asks about an expected finding, not necessarily an abnormal one.

75. While performing an initial assessment on a term neonate with an Asian mother, a bluish marking is observed across the neonate's lower back. What does this finding signify?

1. It's probably a sign of birth trauma.
2. It's probably a telangiectatic hemangioma.
3. It's probably a typical marking in dark-skinned races.
4. It probably indicates that hyperbilirubinemia may follow.

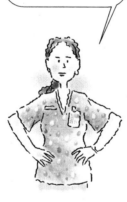

Your role as a preceptor is to help "mold" future nurses.

76. A nurse in the neonate nursery is serving as preceptor for a student nurse. The student asks the nurse why a neonate's head is cone-shaped. Which response is accurate?

1. "It results from caput succedaneum. The difficult labor caused bruising and swelling of the neonate's head."
2. "It results from molding. Overriding of the cranial sutures allows the neonate's head to pass though the birth canal."
3. "It results from cephalohematoma. Some blood has collected between the skull bone and periosteum."
4. "It results from hydrocephalus. Either too much cerebrospinal fluid (CSF) is being formed, or too little is being absorbed."

74. 4. Neonatal skin thickens with maturity and is typically peeling by postterm. Lanugo disappears as pregnancy progresses, with very little remaining on the postterm neonate. Because sole creases increase in number and depth with gestational age, a postterm neonate would have deep sole creases. A postterm neonate would have a well-developed breast bud of 5 to 10 mm in diameter.

CN: Health promotion and maintenance; CNS: None; CL: Analysis

75. 3. This is a Mongolian spot, commonly found over the lumbosacral area in neonates of Black, Asian, Latin American, or Native American origin. The coloration is due to the deposition of melanocytes, not erythrocytes, and, without other findings, isn't a bruise resulting from a birth trauma. A telangiectatic hemangioma is a salmon pink coloration found at the nape of the neck, eyelids, and forehead. A Mongolian spot is a deep dermal infiltration of melanocytes, so there would be no breakdown of erythrocytes to cause hyperbilirubinemia.

CN: Health promotion and maintenance; CNS: None; CL: Analysis

76. 2. Molding refers to overlapping of the cranial sutures, which causes the neonate's head to appear cone-shaped. Caput succedaneum, cephalohematoma, and hydrocephalus don't result in a cone-shaped head. Caput succedaneum is an area of localized swelling and bruising over a presenting part. Cephalohematoma is a collection of blood between the skull bone and periosteum. Hydrocephalus is an increase in the size of the entire head as a result of increased CSF volume.

CN: Health promotion and maintenance; CNS: None; CL: Analysis

CN: Client needs category   CNS: Client needs subcategory   CL: Cognitive level

77. A neonate receiving formula feedings is discharged from the neonate nursery. Twenty-four hours later, the mother calls the hospital, stating that the neonate is vomiting most of his feedings. Which statement by the mother indicates that she needs further discharge instructions?

　　1. "Every time I feed him, he spits up about a teaspoonful of formula onto his bib."
　　2. "I'm using prepared formula, and he takes ½ oz to 1 oz every 3 to 4 hours."
　　3. "I feed him every time he cries. Sometimes he eats 4 oz at a time every couple of hours."
　　4. "I burp him after each ½ oz of formula."

78. A healthy term neonate born by cesarean delivery was admitted to the transitional nursery 30 minutes ago and placed under a radiant warmer. The neonate has an axillary temperature of 99.5° F (37.5° C), a respiratory rate of 80 breaths/minute, and a heelstick glucose value of 60 mg/dl. Which action should the nurse take?

　　1. Wrap the neonate warmly and place him in an open crib.
　　2. Administer an oral glucose feeding of dextrose 10% in water.
　　3. Increase the temperature setting on the radiant warmer.
　　4. Obtain an order for I.V. fluid administration.

79. A home health nurse assesses a neonate who is 48 hours old and was discharged from the hospital 24 hours ago. Which assessment finding indicates a potential problem?

　　1. The neonate cries but no tears appear.
　　2. Small papules appear all over the neonate's skin.
　　3. The neonate doesn't turn his head in the direction that his cheek is stroked.
　　4. The neonate produces a greenish brown stool.

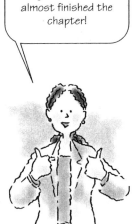

You're doing great! You've almost finished the chapter!

77. 3. Feeding the neonate every time he cries results in overfeeding. A neonate's crying doesn't always signal hunger; sometimes it means his diaper is wet, he needs to suck, or he wants to be held. A neonate who's spitting up should be burped after every ounce of formula or less. For the first few days, the neonate's normal stomach capacity is 15 ml, so he should be fed every 3 to 4 hours. All neonates spit up a small amount because of an immature cardiac sphincter.

CN: Physiological integrity; CNS: Basic care and comfort; CL: Application

78. 4. Assessment findings indicate that the neonate is in respiratory distress—most likely from transient tachypnea, which is common after cesarean delivery. The normal respiratory rate is 30 to 60 breaths/minute; a neonate with a rate of 80 breaths/minute shouldn't be fed but should receive I.V. fluids until the respiratory rate returns to normal. To allow close observation for worsening respiratory distress, the neonate should be kept unclothed in the radiant warmer. Temperature is in the normal range; raising the warmer's temperature setting would cause overheating and worsen the neonate's respiratory distress.

CN: Physiological integrity; CNS: Basic care and comfort; CL: Application

79. 3. A normal, healthy neonate turns in the direction that the cheek is stroked. Failure to do so may indicate a neurologic problem, which the nurse should report to the physician. A neonate's lacrimal glands are immature, resulting in tearless crying for up to 2 months. Erythema toxicum neonatorum causes a transient maculopapular rash—a normal finding in all neonates. Greenish brown stools at 48 hours are normal and indicate that the neonate is eliminating formula or breast milk instead of meconium.

CN: Health promotion and maintenance; CNS: None; CL: Application

80. A nurse is administering vitamin K (AquaMEPHYTON) to a preterm neonate following delivery. The medication comes in a concentration of 2 mg/ml, and the ordered dose is 0.5 mg to be given subcutaneously. How many milliliters should the nurse administer? Record your answer using two decimal points.

_____milliliters

80. 0.25. Use the following formula to calculate drug dosages: Dose on hand/Quantity on hand = Dose desired/X. Plug in the values and the equation is as follows: 2 mg/ml = 0.5 mg/X. X = 0.25 ml.

CN: Physiological integrity; CNS: Pharmacological and parenteral therapies; CL: Application

81. A nurse is eliciting reflexes in a neonate during a physical examination. Identify the area the nurse would touch to elicit a plantar grasp reflex.

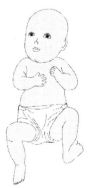

81. To elicit a plantar grasp reflex, the nurse should touch the sole of the foot near the base of the digits, causing flexion or grasping. This reflex disappears around age 9 months.

CN: Health promotion and maintenance; CNS: None; CL: Application

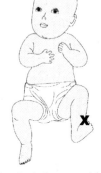

82. What information should a nurse include when teaching postcircumcision care to parents of a neonate prior to discharge from the hospital? Select all that apply:
1. The infant must void before being discharged.
2. Petroleum jelly should be applied to the glans of the penis with each diaper change.
3. The infant can take tub baths while the circumcision heals.
4. Any blood noted on the front of the diaper should be reported.
5. The circumcision will require care for 2 to 4 days after discharge.

82. 1, 2, 5. It's necessary for the infant to void prior to discharge to ensure that the urethra isn't obstructed. A lubricating ointment is appropriate and is applied with each diaper change. Typically, the penis heals within 2 to 4 days, and circumcision care is required for that period only. To prevent infection, avoid giving the infant tub baths until the circumcision is healed; sponge baths are appropriate. A small amount of bleeding is expected following a circumcision; parents should report only a large amount of bleeding.

CN: Health promotion and maintenance; CNS: None; CL: Application

CN: Client needs category   CNS: Client needs subcategory   CL: Cognitive level

Selected references

Anatomy & Physiology Made Incredibly Easy, 3rd ed. Philadelphia: Lippincott Williams & Wilkins, 2009.

Assessment Made Incredibly Easy, 4th ed. Philadelphia: Lippincott Williams & Wilkins, 2008.

Baranoski, S., and Ayello, E.A. *Wound Care Essentials: Practice Principles,* 2nd ed. Philadelphia: Lippincott Williams & Wilkins, 2008.

Bickley, L.S., and Szilagyi, P.G. *Bates' Guide to Physical Examination and History Taking,* 10th ed. Philadelphia: Lippincott Williams & Wilkins, 2009.

Bowden, V.R., and Greenberg, C.S. *Pediatric Nursing Procedures,* 2nd ed. Philadelphia: Lippincott Williams & Wilkins, 2008.

Boyd, M.A. *Psychiatric Nursing: Contemporary Practice,* 4th ed. Philadelphia: Lippincott Williams & Wilkins, 2008.

Cardiovascular Care Made Incredibly Easy, 2nd ed. Philadelphia: Lippincott Williams & Wilkins, 2009.

ECG Interpretation Made Incredibly Easy, 5th ed. Philadelphia: Lippincott Williams & Wilkins, 2011.

Fauci, A., et al. *Harrison's Principles of Internal Medicine,* 17th ed. New York: McGraw-Hill, 2009.

Fischbach, F., & Dunning, M.B., eds. *A Manual of Laboratory and Diagnostic Tests,* 8th ed. Philadelphia: Lippincott Williams & Wilkins, 2009.

Hockenberry, M.J., and Wilson, D. *Wong's Nursing Care of Infants and Children,* 8th ed. St. Louis: Mosby–Year Book, Inc., 2007.

Ignatavicius, D.D., and Workman, M.L. *Medical-Surgical Nursing: Patient-Centered Collaborative Care,* 6th ed. Philadelphia: Elsevier, 2010.

Judge, N.L. "Neurovascular Assessment," *Nursing Standard* 21(45):39-44, July 2007.

Karch, A.M. *Focus on Nursing Pharmacology,* 5th ed. Philadelphia: Lippincott Williams & Wilkins, 2010.

Kyle, T. *Essentials of Pediatric Nursing.* Philadelphia: Lippincott Williams & Wilkins, 2008.

Lippincott's Nursing Procedures, 5th ed. Philadelphia: Lippincott Williams & Wilkins, 2008.

Nettina, S.M. *Lippincott Manual of Nursing Practice,* 9th ed. Philadelphia: Lippincott Williams & Wilkins, 2010.

Nursing 2010 Drug Handbook. Philadelphia: Lippincott Williams & Wilkins, 2010.

Pillitteri, A. *Maternal & Child Health Nursing: Care of the Childbearing and Childrearing Family,* 6th ed. Philadelphia: Lippincott Williams & Wilkins, 2010.

Porth, C.M., and Matfin, G. *Pathophysiology: Concepts of Altered Health States,* 8th ed. Philadelphia: Lippincott Williams & Wilkins, 2009.

Professional Guide to Diseases, 9th ed. Philadelphia: Lippincott Williams & Wilkins, 2009.

Smeltzer, S.C., et al. *Brunner & Suddarth's Textbook of Medical-Surgical Nursing,* 12th ed. Philadelphia: Lippincott Williams & Wilkins, 2010.

Taylor, C.R., et al. *Fundamentals of Nursing: The Art and Science of Nursing Care,* 6th ed. Philadelphia: Lippincott Williams & Wilkins, 2008.

Townsend, M.C., and Pedersen, D.D. *Essentials of Psychiatric Mental Health Nursing: Concepts of Care in Evidence-Based Practice.* Philadelphia: F.A. Davis Company, 2008.

Wilson, D., and Hockenberry, M.J. *Wong's Clinical Manual of Pediatric Nursing,* 7th ed. St. Louis: Mosby–Year Book, Inc., 2008.

Index

A

Abdomen
  in neonate, 90
Abruptio placentae, 50, 58–59
Acquired immunodeficiency syndrome
  in pregnancy, 24, 34–35
Adolescence
  pregnancy in, 24, 35–36
Alpha fetoprotein, 31
Amniocentesis, 31–32
Amnioinfusion, 61
Amnion, 30
Amniotic fluid, 31
Amniotic fluid embolism, 50, 59
Amniotomy, 70
Anesthesia, during labor and
      delivery, 57
Ankle edema, during pregnancy, 29
Antepartum care, 493–518
  client care on, 24–26, 34–44
  diagnostic tests in, 31–34
  discomforts of pregnancy, 29
  estimating delivery dates and
        gestational age, 28
  fetal development and
        structures, 29–31
  key concepts, 23
  normal antepartum period, 23–28
  practice questions on, 44–48
Apgar scoring, 88, 89t

B

Backache, during pregnancy, 29
Biophysical profile, 33
Birth, emergency, 51, 66–68
Blood type
  in pregnancy, 31
Braxton Hicks contractions, 23, 49
Breast-feeding
  instructions for, 94
Breasts
  postpartum, 76
  in pregnancy, 29
Breath, shortness of, in pregnancy, 29

C

Cardiovascular system
  labor and, 54
  in neonate, 85
  postpartum, 73
  pregnancy and, 23, 26
Cesarean birth, 67
Chadwick's sign, 23
Chest in neonate, 90
Chorion, 30
Chorionic villi sampling, 32
Circulation
  after delivery, 73
  in fetus, 31
Circumcision, care after, 94
Client needs, 12
  categories of, 3, 5t
Client safety, 12
Coagulation studies
  in pregnancy, 31
Computer testing, 4–6
Conception, 29–30
Constipation, pregnancy and, 29
Contractions, uterine, 49, 54

D

Dehydration in pregnancy, 54
Delegation, 13–14
Delivery date, estimating, 28
Depression, postpartum, 73, 79–80
Diabetes mellitus
  in pregnancy, 24, 36–37
Dilation, 53
Disseminated intravascular coagulation
  during labor and delivery, 50, 60
Doll's eye reflex, 90
Down syndrome, 31
Drug dependency, in neonate, 86, 93–95
Dystocia, 50–51, 60–61

E

Ears
  in neonate, 90
Eclampsia, 25, 41

(continued)

Ectoderm, 30
Ectopic pregnancy, 24, 37–38
Effacement, 53
Effleurage, 57
Electrolyte balance
  labor and, 54
Emergency birth and preterm labor, 66–69
Endocrine system
  postpartum, 73
  pregnancy and, 27
Endoderm, 30
Episiotomy, 77
Erythroblastosis fetalis, 31
Extrauterine life, adaptations to, 85, 88
Eyes
  in neonate, 90

F

False labor, 49
Fatigue, during pregnancy, 29
Fertilization, 29–30
Fetal alcohol syndrome, 86, 91–92
Fetal blood flow studies, 33
Fetal blood sampling, 57–58
Fetal circulation, 31
Fetal development, 29–31
Fetal distress, 51, 61–62
Fetal heart rate, 32, 55
Fetal lung maturity, 32
Fetal monitoring, 55
Fetal movement count, 34
Fetal position, during labor, 53
Fetus, evaluation of, during labor, 55
Fluid balance
  labor and, 54
Fontanel, 89–90
Fundus, postpartum, 75
  assessment and massage of, 76

G

Gametogenesis, 29
Gastrointestinal system
  labor and, 54
  in neonate, 85

t refers to table

postpartum, 73
pregnancy and, 27
Genital cultures, in pregnancy, 31
Genitalia
in neonate, 90
Genitourinary system
postpartum, 73
pregnancy and, 28
Gestational age, estimating, 28, 32
Gestational hypertension, 25, 41
Gestational trophoblastic disease, 39
Gestation, multiple, 42
Goodell's sign, 23

H

Heartburn, during pregnancy, 29
Heart disease
pregnancy and, 25, 38–39
Hegar's sign, 23
HELLP syndrome, 41, 47
Hematologic studies
in pregnancy, 31
Hematopoietic system
labor and, 54
in neonate, 88
Hemorrhage
postpartum, 74, 78–79, 83, 84
Hemorrhoids, during pregnancy, 29
Hepatic system, in neonate, 88
Hip replacement, 14
Human immunodeficiency virus, in neonate,
86, 92–93
Hydatidiform mole, 25, 39
Hyperbilirubinemia, 31
Hyperemesis gravidarum, 25, 40
Hypertensive disorders
of pregnancy, 25–26, 40–42
Hypospadias, 90
Hypothermia, in neonate, 86, 93

I

Immune system
in neonate, 85, 88
Immunologic studies
in pregnancy, 31
Implantation, 30
Indomethacin, during preterm labor, 68
Infection
neonatal, 87, 95–96
puerperal, 74, 80–81
Insomnia
during pregnancy, 29
Integumentary system, pregnancy
and, 27–28

Internal electronic fetal monitoring, 55
International nurses, guidelines for, 4
Intrapartum care
client care in, 58–66
diagnostic tests in, 57–58
emergency birth and preterm labor,
66–69
key concepts, 49–57
practice questions for, 69–72
Inverted uterus, 51, 62

J

Jaundice, neonatal, 87, 96–97

L

Labor and delivery
components of, 49, 53
evaluating fetus during, 55
evaluating mother during, 53–54
maternal responses to, 54
nursing care during, 56
pain relief during, 56–57
physiological changes after, 73
precipitate, 52, 63–64
preliminary signs of, 49, 53
preterm, 52, 68–69
stages of, 55–56
true *versus* false, 53t
Laboratory values, normal, 14
Laceration, during labor and delivery, 51–52,
62–63
Lamaze breathing, 57
Leg cramps, during pregnancy, 29
Letting-go phase, pregnancy, 75
Leukorrhea, 29
Liver
in neonate, 88
Local infiltration, in labor and delivery, 57
Lochia, 76, 84
Lumbar epidural anesthesia, in labor and
delivery, 57

M

Magnesium sulfate, during preterm
labor, 69
Maslow's hierarchy, 11–12
Mastitis, 74, 77–78
McDonald's rule, 28
Mesoderm, 30
Metabolic system, pregnancy and, 27
Methylergonovine, after delivery, 81
Mouth
in neonate, 90
Multifetal pregnancy, 26, 42–43

N

Nägele's rule, 28
Nausea and vomiting, during
pregnancy, 29
NCLEX
alternate formats for, 6–7
creative studying for, 18–19
maintaining concentration for, 16–17
practice questions for, 20
preparing for, 3–14
sample questions for, 8–10
strategies for success in, 15–20
structure of, 3
study preparations for, 15–16
study schedule, 17–18
Neck, in neonate, 90
Neonatal care
assessment in, 88–91
complications in, 91–98
key concepts in, 85, 88
parent teaching for, 94
practice questions for, 99–102
Neonatal drug dependency, 86, 93–95
Neonatal infections, 87, 95–96
Neonatal jaundice, 87, 96–97
Neonatal skin, 90–91
Neonate
assessment of, 88–91
drug dependency in, 86, 93–95
fetal alcohol syndrome in, 86, 91–92
human immunodeficiency virus in, 86,
92–93
hypothermia in, 86, 93
infections in, 87, 95–96
jaundice in, 87, 88, 96–97
respiratory distress syndrome in,
87, 97–98
tracheoesophageal fistula in, 87, 98
Neural tube defects, 31
Neurosensory system, in neonate, 88
Nipple stimulation stress test, 33
Nonstress test, 32–33
Nose
in neonate, 90
Nursing process, 11
Nutrition, pregnancy and, 28

O

Opioids, in labor and delivery, 57
Oxytocin challenge test, 33

P

Pain relief, during labor and delivery, 56–57
Paracervical block, 57

t refers to table

Percutaneous umbilical blood sampling, 34
Phototherapy, for neonatal jaundice, 97
Physical examination, neonatal, 89–91
Placenta, 56
    formation of, 30
Placenta previa, 26, 43–44
Positive signs of pregnancy, 23
Postpartum care
    assessment in, 75–77
    complications in, 77–81
    key concepts in, 73, 75
    practice questions for, 81–84
Postpartum hemorrhage, 74, 78–79
Precipitate labor, 52, 63–64
Preeclampsia, 25, 41–42
Pregnancy
    acquired immunodeficiency syndrome
        in, 24, 34–35
    adolescent, 24, 35–36
    and delivery date, 28
    diabetes mellitus in, 24, 36–37
    ectopic, 24, 37–38
    fatigue during, 29
    and gestational age, 28
    heart disease in, 25, 38–39
    hypertension in, 25–26, 40–42
    insomnia during, 29
    leg cramps during, 29
    managing discomforts of, 29
    multifetal, 26, 42–43
    normal antepartum period for, 23–28
    nutritional needs during, 28
    physiologic adaptations during, 23, 26
    psychological changes after, 73, 75
    signs and symptoms, 23
    weight gain in, 27
Premature rupture of membranes, 52, 64

Pressure-sensitive catheter, 55
Presumptive signs of pregnancy, 23
Probable signs of pregnancy, 23
Psychological maladaptation, postpartum,
    74, 79–80
Pudendal block, 57
Puerperal infection, 74, 80–81

Q

Questions, alternate-format, 6–10, 14
    key strategies for, 11
Quickening, 23, 28

R

Reflexes, in neonate, 91
Renal system
    labor and, 54
    in neonate, 85
Reproductive system, postpartum, 73
Respiratory distress syndrome, 87, 97–98
Respiratory system
    labor and, 54
    in neonate, 85
    pregnancy and, 27
Rh blood type, 31

S

Skin
    in neonate, 90–91
Spina bifida, 31
Spinal anesthesia, in labor and delivery, 57
Spine, in neonate, 90
Station, fetal, 54
Studying, successful strategies for, 15–20

T

Taking-hold phase, pregnancy, 75
Taking-in phase, pregnancy, 75

Terbutaline, for preterm labor, 46
Therapeutic communication, 12–13
Thermogenesis, neonatal, 85
Tocolytic agents, for preterm labor, 69
Tocotransducer, 55
Tracheoesophageal fistula
    in neonate, 87, 98
Triple screen, 31

U

Ultrasonography, during pregnancy, 32
Umbilical cord, 30, 94
    prolapsed, 52, 65
Urinary frequency, during pregnancy, 29
Urine test
    in pregnancy, 31
Uterine atony, 74, 79
Uterine contractions, 49, 54
Uterine rupture, 53–54, 65–66
Uteroplacental insufficiency, 33
Uterus, inverted, 51, 62

V

Vascular system, after delivery, 73
Vibroacoustic stimulation, 33

W

Weight gain, pregnancy and, 27

Z

Zidovudine, during pregnancy, 92
Zygote, 30